Anesthesiology Applied Exam Board Review

Anesthesiology Applied Exam Board Review

Edited by
Ruchir Gupta, MD
Associate Professor of Anesthesiology
Stony Brook School of Medicine
Stony Brook, NY

Minh Chau Joe Tran, MD
Director, Simulation Training
Department of Anesthesiology
Loma Linda University School of Medicine
Loma Linda, CA

OXFORD
UNIVERSITY PRESS

OXFORD
UNIVERSITY PRESS

Oxford University Press is a department of the University of Oxford. It furthers the University's objective of excellence in research, scholarship, and education by publishing worldwide. Oxford is a registered trade mark of Oxford University Press in the UK and certain other countries.

Published in the United States of America by Oxford University Press
198 Madison Avenue, New York, NY 10016, United States of America.

CIP data is on file at the Library of Congress
ISBN 978–0–19–085247–4

Contents

Contributors

Molly Amin, MD
Department of Anesthesiology
Rutgers New Jersey Medical School
Newark, NJ

Xiaodong Bao, MD, PhD
Department of Anesthesia, Critical Care, and Pain Medicine
Massachusetts General Hospital
Boston, MA

Edouard Belotte, MD
Department of Anesthesiology
Queens Hospital Center
Mount Sinai Hospital
Queens, NY

Monique Cadogan, MD
Department of Anesthesiology
Valley Children's Hospital
Madera, CA

John Cooley, MD
Acting Chairman
Department of Anesthesiology
Westchester Medical Center
Westchester, NY

Shimon Frankel, MD
Department of Anesthesiology
Saint Barnabas Medical Center
Livingston, NJ

Michal Gajewski, DO
Department of Anesthesiology
New Jersey Medical School
Rutgers, The State University of New Jersey
Newark, NJ

Sheryl Glassman, DO
Department of Anesthesiology
Crozer-Keystone Health System
Darby, PA

Anita Gupta, DO
Medical Director
Division of Pain Medicine
Hahnemann University Hospital and Drexel
University College of Medicine
Philadelphia, PA

Ruchir Gupta, MD
Associate Professor of Anesthesiology
Stony Brook School of Medicine
Stony Brook, NY

Sana Na Javeed, MD
Department of Anesthesiology
Stony Brook University Medical Center
Stony Brook, NY

Aimee Kakascik, DO
Department of Anesthesiology
Baylor College of Medicine
Texas Children's Hospital
Houston, TX

Kseniya Khmara, MD
Department of Anesthesiology
Stony Brook University Medical Center
Stony Brook, NY

Ethan Kim, MD
Department of Anesthesiology
Stony Brook University
Medical Center
Stony Brook, NY

Anna Kogan, DO
Department of Anesthesiology
Stony Brook University
Medical Center
Stony Brook, NY

Dieman La, MD
Loma Linda University School
of Medicine
Loma Linda, CA

Sarah Madison, MD
Department of Anesthesiology
Stanford Health
Stanford, CA

Joseph Marino, MD
Department of Anesthesiology
Northwell Hospital Center –
Franklin Hospital
Valley Stream, NY

Dion M. McCall, MD
Department of Anesthesiology
New Jersey Medical School
Rutgers, The State University of
New Jersey
Newark, NJ

Julio Olaya, MD
Department of Anesthesiology
Arkansas Children's Hospital
Little Rock, Arkansas

Frederico Osorio, MD
Anesthesia Consultants of Dallas
Dallas, TX

Sergey Pisklakov, MD
Department of Anesthesiology
Albert Einstein College of Medicine
Bronx, NY
Rutgers New Jersey Medical School
Newark, NJ

Alec C. Runyon, MD
Department of Anesthesiology
Loma Linda University
Medical Center
Loma Linda, CA

Mark Slomovits, MD
Department of Anesthesiology
Hofstra-NSLIJ School of
Medicine
New York, NY

Minh Chau Joe Tran, MD
Department of Anesthesiology
Loma Linda University School of
Medicine
Loma Linda, CA

Barbara Vickers, MD
Department of Anesthesiology
Johns Hopkins University
Hospital
Baltimore, MD

William Vuong, MD
Department of Anesthesiology
Stony Brook University
Medical Center
Stony Brook, NY

Nicholas Weber, DO
IHC-Wheaton Anesthesia
Milwaukee, WI

Peggy Wingard, MD
Department of Anesthesiology
Texas Children's Hospital
Houston, TX

Carl Ying, MD
Department of Anesthesiology
Loma Linda University School of
Medicine
Loma Linda, CA

Stanley Yuan, MD
Virginia Mason Medical Center
Seattle, WA

Introduction

The anesthesia board exam in most parts of the world is typically divided into two parts: a written multiple-choice exam and an oral exam in which a clinical scenario is presented and questions are asked by the examiner related to the stem.

As of 2018, in the United States the oral exam has been enveloped into a larger exam, known as the "applied exam." The applied exam consists of two components: the traditional oral exam and a newer "objective structure clinical exam" (OSCE). For the traditional oral exam, the student has two sessions: a Part 1 session with a long stem, in which the student is asked questions regarding the intraoperative and postoperative care, and a Part 2 session in which the student is given a slightly shorter stem and asked preoperative and intraoperative questions. As an examinee, you will have a short amount of time to review and "dissect" your stem before entering the examination room. Upon entering the exam room, you will find two individuals sitting behind a desk who will ask the questions. At the end of each stem you will be given three short "additional topics" scenarios and four to five questions per scenario. These additional topics are often harder than the main stems because you have no time to review and "dissect" the clinical scenario and the questions asked can be preoperative, intraoperative, or postoperative.

For the OSCE portion of the exam, the student is required to demonstrate proficiency in three out of nine stations. Because the student does not know which three he or she will be tested on, it is imperative to have proficiency in all nine stations.

How to Approach the Applied Exam

The applied exam was not created to merely test knowledge. Successful completion of the written exam attests to the fact that you have sufficient knowledge. Rather, it is meant to determine if you can adequately discuss anesthesia as a trained consultant. The Board wants you to describe everything you do. For example, if asked how you would induce an ASA 1 patient for a cholecystectomy, you cannot say "propofol." You must begin by saying, "After preoxygenating with 100% oxygen and ensuring the airway is normal, I would administer fentanyl, lidocaine, propofol, and, after ensuring that I can ventilate, rocuronium."

If the philosophy of the entire exam could be summed up in one word, it would be *why*. *What* you do is not as important as *why* you do it, so you must give an explanation for your decision. In doing so, it is advisable that you use the term *risks outweighing benefits* or vice versa. Consider the following example:

> Question: Would you administer propofol to a patient with severe CAD?
>
> Answer: No, I would not, because the risks of propofol administration in a patient with severe CAD outweigh the benefits. Propofol is a fast-acting drug that can provide rapid intubating conditions. However, it is associated with hypotension, which can decrease the coronary perfusion pressure necessary to perfuse the myocardium. Thus, I would rather choose a more cardiac-stable drug such as etomidate.

Such an answer allows the examiner to follow your thought process and also determine your level of knowledge. Mostly all decisions in anesthesia have a risk/benefit ratio, and discussing this ratio in your answer will impress your examiners.

Not a Comprehensive Review

This exam is not a spectator sport; it's a tackle sport. Neither this book nor any on this topic can, by itself, get you ready for the exam. You must do practice exams! At our course, www.justoralboards.com, we offer practice mock oral exams that provide similar conditions to those in the actual test. Once in the "hot seat," candidates often find their knowledge disappearing within the shroud of anxiety and nervousness. They also find it difficult to organize their thoughts. This book can help you understand how to formulate your answers and which subtopics to keep in mind when you see your stem, but it cannot, by itself, relieve your anxiety or help you organize your thoughts. For this, you must practice, practice, practice!

How to Use This Book

The examiners have certain topics they "love." Within each topic are subtopics that they will inevitably question you on. For example, if your stem is about a patient undergoing a pulmonary lobectomy, you can be certain that the questions they will ask will be about double-lumen tube (DLT) indication/contraindications, diagnosis of placement of DLT placement, management of hypoxia after placement of DLT, among other questions. Knowing what the questions will likely be prior to entering your exam room enables you to formulate your responses and be ready for the questions as they arrive.

Thus, this book is organized into individual chapters of the 32 high-yield exam topics seen on the anesthesia boards. In addition, there are seven additional chapters that contain 10 "additional topics" based on subspecialty. Within each of the 32 high-yield exam topics are the most common subtopics that are tested, and a few questions are provided that are modeled around the subtopics. Most likely, if you have a stem on one of these 32 topics, you will also have questions similar to the ones in the chapter for that topic. Read it! Look at how the answer is formulated! Then, team up with a study partner and test each other using the stems provided to you.

Often candidates will want to practice mock oral exams, but they lack full-length exams with questions AND answers that they can trust to use in testing one another. This book is a solution to that. We encourage the "study buddy" system, and because this book is pocket size, you can carry it around with you during your clinical day and review any exam on your own during your down time.

Learn the Language

As you review for this test, you will realize that this exam has its own unique language. The examiners want you to speak a certain way, using certain terms. As you review the chapters, you will realize how different this language is from the one you speak every day. Many candidates fail every year, not for the lack of knowledge but because they didn't appreciate the jargon and terminology that the anesthesia boards desires. By providing you with answers, this book can help you learn the language. Use it as you move forward with your study.

Format

Each chapter in this book has been written in either the Stem 1 (long form) or Stem 2 (short form) format. Our desire in doing so was to give you the opportunity to practice "dissecting" both types of stems. On the exam, Stem 1 questions will be strictly in the intraoperative and postoperative areas, whereas Stem 2 questions will be preoperative and intraoperative. For your benefit, we have provided questions on preoperative, intraoperative, and postoperative sections for all of the stems, regardless of whether they are Stem 1 or 2. This way, you will be familiar with the major subtopics in each facet of anesthesia care.

Also, the level of difficulty in each exam has purposely been kept at a slightly lower level than the exams you would normally encounter with our course, www.justoralboards.com. This is intentional. We want you to first develop a solid, broad-based foundation by learning about the major high-yield topics for the oral exam. Once you have mastered these high-yield topics, you will be in a good position to start taking more difficult exams, in which multiple topics are combined. For example, perhaps the patient having a pulmonary lobectomy has sickle cell disease. In this book, these topics are covered separately, but once you understand the anesthetic implications of both and what key subtopics the examiner would want to cover in each of these, you are in a better position to begin integrating these concepts.

Finally, have faith in yourself and your abilities as a clinician. If you are studying for the oral exam, you already have a great deal to be proud of. You obviously have a solid knowledge base (which you perhaps forgot by now but can easily relearn) and you completed an anesthesia residency. Thus, you know how to administer anesthesia. Use this book to review what you have already done, and speak to your examiner like you are speaking to a third-year medical student, leaving out no details and being thorough in your response and explanation. Work hard, study hard, and do as many mock orals as you can. Every time you are about to give up, just think how much better you will feel when you click on your exam score and see the word "PASS." Take it from two people who did it the first time around: it's worth all the agony and heartache.

I Oral Examination Cases

1 General: Obesity and Difficult Airway

Ruchir Gupta

A 38-year-old male weighing 190 kg and with a height of 5 feet 6 inches is scheduled for a laparoscopic gastric bypass.

Past medical history: The patient has diabetes mellitus (DM), hypertension (HTN), gastroesophageal reflux disease (GERD), and obstructive sleep apnea (OSA) requiring continuous positive airway pressure (CPAP). His past medical history is also significant for hypertension, severe GERD, hiatal hernia, depression, and OSA requiring CPAP.

Physical exam: Pulse 74 beats per minute (bpm), blood pressure (BP) 130/68 mmHg, respiratory rate (RR) 14, temperature (T) 36°C, 97% on room air (RA). On physical exam, his Mallampati score is 3 and his cervical range of motion is normal. His dentition is intact. Auscultation reveals normal breath sounds bilaterally with regular rate and rhythm.

Electrocardiogram (EKG): Normal sinus rhythm (NSR).

Labs: Serum glucose is 153 mg/dL, otherwise his complete blood count (CBC) and basic chemistry panel are within normal limits.

A. Preoperative Evaluation

Obesity

Question 1

How is body mass index (BMI) calculated?

Answer 1

BMI is calculated by dividing the weight in kilograms (kg) by the height in meters squared (kg/m^2).

Obstructive Sleep Apnea

Question 2

How is obstructive sleep apnea (OSA) different from obstructive sleep hypopnea (OSH)?

Answer 2

OSA is cessation of airflow for more than 10 seconds, five or more times per hour of sleep. There is a >4% decrease in O_2 while the patient is asleep. By contrast, in OSH there is a decrease in airflow of >50% for more than 10 seconds, 15 or more times per hour of sleep. The decrease in O_2 saturation during these episodes is also >4%.

Question 3

How is the definitive diagnosis of OSA made?

Answer 3

Although OSA may be suspected by history, physical examination, and/or comorbidities, a definitive diagnosis requires a formal sleep study.

Question 4

What are the systemic manifestations of OSA?

Answer 4

OSA affects multiple organ systems:

Cardiac—patients usually have hypertension and left ventricular hypertrophy (LVH). Pulmonary HTN may also be present.

Pulmonary—there is increased ventilation/perfusion (V/Q) mismatch from decreased functional residual capacity (FRC) and atelectasis.

Gastrointestinal (GI)—often the stomach is displaced upward because of extra abdominal, placing them at risk for GERD.

Renal—the patient may have hypertensive nephropathy.

Neurological—hypersomnolence is frequently observed with increased sensitivity to anesthetic agents.

Question 5

How is OSA distinguished from the Pickwickian syndrome (PS)?

Answer 5

OSA is defined as cessation of airflow for more than 10 seconds, five or more times per hour of sleep. Pickwickian syndrome is characterized by chronic hypoventilation that is worse during sleep, resulting in an elevation in partial pressure of carbon dioxide ($PaCO_2$) levels. Indeed, the diagnosis of PS is BMI >30, $PaCO_2$ >44 mmHg, and no alternative explanation for hypoventilation. Patients with PS often have coexisting OSA, but not every patient with one disease will necessarily have the other. Patients with PS frequently develop sequelae from the CO_2 retention: polycythemia, cor pulmonale, and somnolence.

Question 6

How does this patient's history of OSA affect your anesthetic management?

Answer 6

Preoperatively, a thorough history and physical examination (H&P) must be done to assess for any comorbid conditions. I would exercise caution in using sedative drugs because of increased sensitivity in OSA patients to central nervous system (CNS) depressants such as midazolam. A thorough airway exam must also be done because most of these patients have an airway that can present difficulties. Intraoperatively, care must be taken to preoxygenate these patients thoroughly as they are prone to rapid desaturation secondary to low FRC. I would also have the difficult-airway cart in the room and consider an awake intubation if the airway was non-reassuring. During the course of the surgery, I would use a multimodal pain management regimen including intravenous (IV) nonsteroidal anti-inflammatory drugs (NSAIDs), IV Tylenol, rectus sheath block, and local wound infiltration to decrease narcotic use. Postoperatively, I would extubate in the head-up position to improve pulmonary mechanics and extubate only after the patient is fully awake. I would also have a CPAP machine ready in the post-anesthesia care unit (PACU) and continue to monitor the patient closely in the PACU for any episodes of apnea and desaturation.

B. Intraoperative Management

Monitors

Question 1

What monitors will you use for this patient?

Answer 1

I would use the standard American Society of Anesthesiologists (ASA) monitors (pulse oximeter, noninvasive blood pressure measurements, a 5-lead EKG, a temperature probe, and a capnograph), a neuromuscular blockade monitor, and if peripheral intravenous (PIV) access is difficult, I would place a central line. I would also ask for a Foley catheter to be placed.

Question 2

The nurse informs you she has a large-sized BP cuff. What do you do?

Answer 2

I could attempt to place a standard-sized BP cuff on the forearm or the lower leg. I could also place a large-sized cuff or, alternatively, an arterial line.

Premedication

Question 3

What premedication, if any, would you give this patient?

Answer 3

To avoid possible respiratory depression in morbidly obese patients with OSA, premedication is used sparingly, if at all. Thus, if the patient was anxious, I would start by reassuring the patient. If the patient was still anxious, then, after monitors have been placed in the operating room, I would administer a low dose of midazolam and/or ketamine. Due to risk of aspiration, I would administer sodium citrate to decrease stomach acidity, and promotility agents such as metoclopromide to enhance gastric emptying.

Intubation

Question 4

How would you intubate this patient?

Answer 4

Based on the information provided, management of the patient's airway may be difficult, and so after preoxygenating the patient with 100% oxygen, I would perform an awake oral fiber-optic intubation. I would topicalize the airway with 1–2% lidocaine spray or nebulizer and perform a superior laryngeal nerve block by injecting 2 mL of 2% lidocaine, just anterior to the cornu of the hyoid bones, and a transtracheal recurrent laryngeal nerve block.

Question 5

Your resident accidently administers a bolus of propofol to the patient to prevent him from moving during the awake fiber-optic intubation AFOI. A few seconds later, the patient becomes apneic and begins to desaturate. What will you do?

Answer 5

I would immediately call for help and perform mask ventilation in an attempt to improve this patient's oxygenation while attempting to awaken the patient.

Question 6

You mask ventilate the patient and obtain some end-tidal carbon dioxide ($EtCO_2$), but the patient continues to desaturate, with an oxygen saturation of 90% and decreasing. Mask ventilation is getting progressively more difficult. What will you do?

Answer 6

I would again call for help if it has not yet arrived and would perform direct laryngoscopy. If that did not work or I was unable to mask ventilate the patient, I would place a laryngeal mask airway (LMA) and ventilate through that device.

Question 7

You successfully place an LMA and the desaturation improves. Should you cancel the case once the patient awakens?

Answer 7

It depends on the status of the patient. If there is a great deal of oral swelling and bleeding secondary to my ventilation and direct laryngoscopy attempts, I would delay this case for a few days until the swelling has subsided. If, however, the oropharynx seemed uninjured and there were no signs of bleeding or swelling, I would reattempt my awake fiber-optic intubation and proceed as scheduled.

Maintenance of Anesthesia

Question 8

The airway is now secured with an endotracheal tube (ETT). What agents will you use to maintain anesthesia?

Answer 8

I would choose short-acting agents to reduce the risk of postoperative sedation. Desflurane is desirable because it is relatively insoluble in fat, has a fast wake-up time, faster return of airway reflexes, and decreased amount of hepatic metabolism. For muscle relaxation, I would choose cisatracurium or rocuronium.

C. Postoperative Care

Extubation

Question 1

Would you extubate this patient? If so, how?

Answer 1

Assuming there were no adverse intraoperative events and significant volume shifts, I would want to extubate this patient immediately at the end of the procedure. I would have emergency airway equipment on standby, place the patient in the sitting position to optimize pulmonary mechanics, ensure the patient has been adequately reversed, and have the patient spontaneously breathing with adequate tidal volumes and a normal respiratory rate. Once the patient was responding to commands and able to protect his airway, I would extubate.

Question 2

What respiratory parameters can be used for extubation?

Answer 2

Respiratory rates between 10 and 30 breaths per minute, peripheral oxygen saturation (SpO_2) greater than 95% on fraction of inspired oxygen (FiO_2) of 0.4, vital capacity greater than 10 mL/kg of ideal body weight (IBW), and tidal volume greater than 5 mL/kg of IBW.

Hyperglycemia

Question 3

The nurse in the PACU pages you to tell you the blood glucose is 253 mg/dL. Why is controlling blood glucose in the perioperative period important?

Answer 3

The consequences of acute hyperglycemia include impaired immune response with increased risk of infection, impaired wound healing, dehydration, and electrolyte disturbances secondary to the osmotic diuretic effect of high serum glucose levels. This diabetic patient, who takes oral hypoglycemic medication, is at risk for developing potentially fatal nonketotic hyperosmolar coma.

Pain Control

Question 4

What is your plan for postoperative pain management in this patient?

Answer 4

I would provide this patient with non-opioid analgesics such as Tylenol and NSAIDs. I would also have asked the surgeon to place local anesthesia around the incisions intraoperatively. In addition, for pain refractory to these medications, patient-controlled analgesia (PCA) can provide relief without risking overdosing as the patient must be awake and alert in order to administer the medicine. Given the presence of OSA I would place this patient in a monitored setting overnight.

Question 5

A colleague suggests the use of patient-controlled epidural analgesia (PCEA) instead of PCA. What are some benefits of PCEA, in comparison to PCA?

Answer 5

The benefit of PCEA over PCA is that less opioid medication is used because local anesthesia can also be delivered epidurally. The lower opioid requirement results in fewer side effects, such as respiratory complications, while also ensuring effective analgesia.

Mental Status Change

Question 6

A few hours later, the PACU nurse informs you that the patient is "disoriented." What is your differential diagnosis?

Answer 6

My differential includes the following:

1. Unstable vital signs: hypoxia, hypotension, malignant arrhythmia
2. Anesthesia-induced causes: residual anesthesia, narcotic overdose or reaction
3. Possible delirium tremens from withdrawal from a previously unknown substance abuse agent
4. Potential metabolic and endocrinological causes: hyponatremia, hypokalemia, hypocalcemia, hypoglycemia, hyperglycemia, hypothermia, hypothyroidism, and Addison's disease, among others
5. Neurological causes include postictal state, cerebral edema, and stroke.

Question 7

How will you respond?

Answer 7

First, I would ensure that the patient is adequately oxygenating and ventilating and the vital signs are stable. Next, I would perform a focused history and physical exam. From the history, I would review the anesthetic record as well as the nurses' notes to see what medications the patient had received, when the symptoms began, whether they were getting worse or better, and what the severity of the disorientation was. During the physical, I would listen for breath sounds and look for neurological signs, including pupillary size and any focal neurological deficits. Finally, I would order stat labs including arterial blood gases (ABG), electrolytes with glucose, and a CBC to evaluate for anemia. If a stroke is suspected, a stat head computed tomography (CT) and neurology consult would be obtained.

Suggested Readings

Barash PG, Cullen BF, Stoelting RK, Cahalan M, Stock CM, eds. *Clinical Anesthesia*. 6th ed. Philadelphia, PA: Lippincott Williams & Wilkins; 2009.

Miller RD, Eriksson LI, Fleisher LA, Wiener-Kornish JP, Young WL, eds. *Miller's Anesthesia*. 7th ed. Philadelphia, PA: Churchill Livingstone Elsevier; 2010.

Yao F, Fontes ML, Malhotra V, eds. *Yao and Artusio's Anesthesiology: Problem-Oriented Patient Management*. 7th ed. Philadelphia, PA: Lippincott Williams & Wilkins; 2011.

2 General: Myasthenia Gravis

Shimon Frankel

Stem 2

A 54-year-old female presents for laparoscopic resection of the colon. The patient has a history of colon cancer and myasthenia gravis for which she is on pyridostigmine and prednisone. Her vital signs are BP 121/55 mmHg, RR 12, HR 64 bpm, room air saturation 99%. Hemoglobin (Hb) = 11.4 g/dL.

A. Preoperative Evaluation

Assessment of Severity

Question 1

1. How would you assess if this patient is optimized for surgery?

Answer 1

I would obtain a focused history and physical. From the history, I would want to know if her disease is limited to ocular muscles or if there is involvement of her extremities or respiratory/laryngeal muscles as evidenced by trouble chewing, swallowing, or talking. I would also want to know if the patient has ever had surgery before, whether she has had any prolonged intubations or problems with anesthesia or any episodes of myasthenic crisis, and whether her symptoms have been stable over the past few weeks. From the physical, I would assess bilateral motor strength in all of her extremities and see if she displays any signs of pharyngeal or respiratory muscle involvement.

Question 2

What is myasthenia gravis (MG)? What other medical conditions is MG closely associated with?

Answer 2

MG is an autoimmune disorder involving antibodies to the α subunit of the postsynaptic nicotinic acetylcholine receptor at the neuromuscular junction leading to a decreased number of functional receptors. With repeated stimulation and decreased acetylcholine release, fatigue occurs. The extent of involvement can be limited to ocular muscles, but muscles of respiration and swallowing can also be involved, causing respiratory distress or aspiration.

MG is occasionally associated with thymus hyperplasia, thymomas, or autoimmune diseases such as thyroid disease, pernicious anemia, and rheumatoid arthritis (RA). MG also occurs in women with certain HLA types.

Question 3

Would you obtain pulmonary functions tests (PFTs)? Why? Why not?

Answer 3

I would not obtain PFTs in this patient unless there was a severe respiratory component as evidenced by the patient's history and physical exam. If the patient had severe respiratory symptoms, negative inspiratory force (NIF) and forced vital capacity (FVC) could be used as a reference to determine optimal conditions for extubation or the need for postoperative mechanical ventilation. They may also help in determining appropriateness for ambulatory surgery. If the patient has a thymoma, flow volume loops (FVLs) can demonstrate the extent of impairment and whether it is fixed or dynamic.

Medication for MG

Question 4

Should the patient continue the morning dose of pyridostigmine on the day of surgery? Why?

Answer 4

Although there is no clear-cut answer to this question, I would recommend continuing the pyridostigmine in order to avoid any possible respiratory difficulties before surgery. The disadvantage of continuing cholinesterase inhibition is the possibility of prolonged motor block with succinylcholine, and the possibility of developing a cholinergic crisis.

Question 5

Why is this patient on corticosteroids?

Answer 5

MG is an autoimmune disease. Corticosteroids suppress the immune system and attenuate the production of these abnormal autoantibodies to the acetylcholine receptors at the motor endplate. Treatment of MG usually begins with cholinesterase inhibitors. For more advanced disease, corticosteroids and thymectomy are used. In more severe cases, immunosuppressants (such as azathioprine or cyclosporine) and plasmapheresis are used. Intravenous immunoglobulin (IVIG) is used for myasthenic crisis.

Question 6

Would you administer preoperative steroids? Why? Why not?

Answer 6

Yes, I would administer a stress dose of steroids, hydrocortisone 100 mg every 8 hours on the day of surgery and then taper it postoperatively. Patients taking chronic glucocorticoids may have suppressed adrenal function. Thus, I would continue her chronic dose perioperatively and be alert for signs of adrenal insufficiency.

Question 7

Would you sedate this patient preoperatively?

Answer 7

If there is a question as to her respiratory reserve I would avoid sedative premedication. If the symptoms are primarily ocular, a small dose of a benzodiazepine would be acceptable, especially since emotional stress could exacerbate myasthenia.

Question 8

Is there anything you would tell this patient about her postoperative course?

Answer 8

I would inform the patient and family that symptoms may worsen perioperatively but will usually return to baseline. I would also mention the possibility of postoperative mechanical ventilation.

Lambert-Eaton Syndrome

Question 9

What is Lambert-Eaton myasthenic syndrome (LEMS)?

Answer 9

This is a disease of motor weakness that is often characterized by proximal limb weakness, especially of the lower extremities. It is caused by autoantibodies to the voltage-gated calcium channels of the presynaptic membrane. Calcium is not able to enter the nerve ending and to allow acetylcholine release. Weakness typically improves with repetitive use as this allows for buildup of calcium, allowing for acetylcholine release. Patients are sensitive to both depolarizing and nondepolarizing muscle relaxants and patients may need postoperative respiratory support.

LEMS is often seen as a paraneoplastic syndrome related to small-cell cancer of the lung. It may also be seen with sarcoidosis, other malignancies, thyroiditis, and collagen vascular diseases.

B. Intraoperative Management

Anesthesia

Question 1

Would you select a general or a regional technique for this patient?

Answer 1

Assuming there are no contraindications, I would prefer a regional anesthetic technique for this case because it avoids muscle relaxation, instrumenting of the airway, and the need for postoperative ventilator support. Patients with MG are usually more resistant to succinylcholine and more sensitive to nondepolarizing muscle relaxants (NDMRs).

Question 2

If you decide on a regional technique, would you select a spinal or an epidural approach?

Answer 2

I would select a continuous epidural approach because it would allow me to run a constant infusion if the operation runs longer than was originally planned. Additionally, it allows me to administer local anesthetics and narcotics postoperatively for pain.

Induction

Question 3

How would you induce general anesthesia in this patient if she refuses a regional technique?

Answer 3

Assuming the patient has a normal airway, I would preoxygenate with 100% oxygen and perform a slow, controlled induction with short-acting agents such as remifentanil, lidocaine, and propofol.

Question 4

The surgeon says he will need muscle relaxation for the case. How do you respond?

Answer 4

I would try to avoid muscle relaxants if possible because even patients with minimal disease may have increased sensitivity to NDMRs. Additionally, inhalational agents often provide adequate muscle relaxation in myasthenic patients to perform surgery. If needed, I would use intermediate-acting muscle relaxants in increments of 0.1–0.2 times the ED95.

Question 5

How would your induction technique change if the patient were at high risk of aspiration?

Answer 5

I would perform a rapid-sequence intubation using succinylcholine at a dose of 1.5–2 mg/kg. Patients with MG are resistant to succinylcholine, but at higher doses it should provide rapid intubating conditions.

Muscle Relaxation

Question 6

Would you use a nerve stimulator during the case? Why or why not?

Answer 6

Yes, I would, but I would bear in mind that it may not be reliable in myasthenic patients because the distribution of muscle weakness is often uneven and many patients may exhibit fade even in the preoperative period.

Question 7

What is the impact of preoperative cholinesterase inhibitor administration on neuromuscular blockade and reversal?

Answer 7

Preoperative pyridostigmine inhibits plasma cholinesterase, and succinylcholine may cause a prolonged block. Reversal of residual nondepolarizing neuromuscular blockade at the end of surgery may be unsuccessful because acetylcholinesterase is already maximally inhibited.

C. Postoperative Care

Postoperative Weakness

Question 1

Are you going to extubate this patient at the end of the case?

Answer 1

It depends on how the case went and whether the patient is meeting extubation criteria. I would not extubate if more than minimal doses of nondepolarizing muscle blocking agents or narcotics were used since the patient may not recover respiratory function immediately.

Question 2

You receive a call from the PACU complaining that the patient is feeling weak. What do you think? What will you do?

Answer 2

Many factors could cause postoperative weakness in a patient with MG. My differentials would include residual muscle relaxant, narcotic overdose, residual inhalational anesthetic, myasthenic crisis, cholinergic crisis, hypothermia, hypocarbia, and acidosis.

I would assess the patient's vital signs, saturation, and respiratory pattern. If the patient was showing signs of respiratory insufficiency, I would reintubate her. If she was stable, I would look for the cause of her weakness, review the anesthetic record, and consider a tensilon test to evaluate if she was in myasthenic crisis or cholinergic crisis. With myasthenic crisis, her symptoms should improve with edrophonium; with cholinergic crisis, they would not.

Crisis

Question 3

What is a myasthenic crisis? What are the precipitating factors?

Answer 3

A myasthenic crisis, which implies severe bulbar or respiratory symptoms, can be precipitated by progression of disease or other factors. Some factors that may worsen symptoms are infection, recent surgery, emotional stress, and interruption of immunosuppressants. Drugs associated with worsening symptoms include aminoglycosides, polymyxins, fluoroquinolones, clindamycin, anticonvulsants, beta blockers, calcium channel blockers, corticosteroids, local anesthetics, magnesium, ketamine, neuromuscular blockers, and anticholinergics. Hypothermia, acidosis, and electrolyte abnormalities such as hypokalemia or hypermagnesemia can compound the severe muscle weakness.

Question 4

What is a cholinergic crisis? How would you treat a patient with a cholinergic crisis?

Answer 4

A cholinergic crisis occurs when the patient is overdosed with cholinesterase inhibitors and may show symptoms such as excessive salivation, sweating, abdominal cramps, urinary urgency, bradycardia, muscle fasciculations, or muscle weakness. The treatment is supportive and includes endotracheal intubation, atropine, and cessation of cholinesterase inhibitors until the crisis is over.

Question 5

What is your plan for postoperative pain? Are there any special considerations?

Answer 5

Ideally, I would use intrathecal morphine because this can provide prolonged pain control with less respiratory depression than intravenous morphine. If that is not an option, I would use intravenous narcotics sparingly with NSAIDs and acetaminophen as adjuncts. If an epidural or intercostal nerve block were used, I would avoid ester local anesthetics because they are metabolized by plasma cholinesterase and can worsen symptoms. Instead, I would use amide local anesthetics in reduced doses.

Suggested Readings

Abel M, Eisenkraft JB. Anesthetic implications of myasthenia gravis. *Mt Sinai J Med.* 2002;69(1-2):31–37.

Blichfeldt-Lauridsen L, Hansen BD. Anesthesia and myasthenia gravis. *Acta Anaesthesiol Scand.* 2012;56:17–22.

Miller RD, Eriksson LI, Fleisher LA, Wiener-Kronish JP, eds. *Miller's Anesthesia.* 7th ed. Philadelphia, PA: Churchill Livingstone; 2009.

3 General: Laryngeal Papillomatosis

Aimee Kakascik

Stem 1

A 12-year-old, 55 kg male from Nigeria is to have surgical excision and ablation of laryngeal papillomas.

History of present illness: The patient has had the diagnosis since early childhood as the human papilloma virus was transmitted to the child during pregnancy. He has had surgical treatments every 6 to 9 weeks since he was 2 years old. He presents today as usual with a soft, hoarse voice and stridor. He is able to go to school but is unable to participate in any sports or physical education classes.

Past medical history: His medical history is otherwise negative except he is positive for human immunodeficiency virus (HIV).

Medications: He takes cidofovir and interferon.

Physical exam: vital signs: BP 130/78 mmHg, P 105 bpm, RR = 22, room air (RA) saturation 97%.

General: He is anxious about the procedure.

Airway: Mallampati class 2, no loose teeth.

Cardiovascular: Regular rate and rhythm (RRR).

Lungs: clear to ausculation (CTA) bilaterally.

Labs: Hematocrit (Hct) = 31%, platelets = 250 K, Na = 135 mEq/L, K = 4.1 mEq/L.

A. Preoperative Evaluation

Respiratory

Question 1

Do you need any additional studies to evaluate the patient's airway?

Answer 1

In reviewing his last anesthetic record and confirming with the otolaryngologist that his condition is not worse than before, I would also be interested in any imaging studies such as a neck CT, which can help me determine the size, shape, and location of the lesion.

Question 2

Would you want pulmonary function tests?

Answer 2

No. Based on the history given, it appears that the patient has had obstruction at the larynx for years. Thus, a thorough H&P would provide the best information for the management of this child.

Question 3

What would a flow-volume loop of this child look like?

Answer 3

The flow-volume loop would show flattening of the inspiratory limb, suggesting variable extrathoracic upper airway obstruction or flattening of both the inspiratory and expiratory limbs if the upper airway obstruction is fixed.

Cardiac

Question 4

Do you have any cardiovascular concerns regarding this patient? If so, how would you address them?

Answer 4

Yes. My concern is that given his long-standing chronic airway obstruction, there is potential for development of right ventricular hypertrophy and cor pulmonale. I would want a baseline EKG and echocardiogram to determine the presence and extent of any cardiac remodeling that may have occurred in response to the chronic airway obstruction.

Question 5

What would the EKG of a patient with cor pulmonale show?

Answer 5

Right atrial hypertrophy would be seen by peaked P waves in leads II, III, and aVF. Right ventricular hypertrophy would be seen by right-axis deviation and a partial or complete right bundle branch block.

Premedication

Question 6

Would you give any preoperative medication for anxiolysis?

Answer 6

Yes, I would give PO midazolam with supplemental oxygen while the child is on telemetry if a preoperative reassuring visit was not enough.

Question 7

Would you start a peripheral intravenous line before or after induction?

Answer 7

If the patient was comfortable with having an IV line placed, I would place it before induction. If the patient is fearful of needles, I would place it after induction to decrease agitation and increased oxygen demand with airway obstruction.

B. Intraoperative Management

Induction

Question 1

How would you induce the patient?

Answer 1

If the child does not have an IV in place, I would perform a slow inhalational induction with sevoflurane and 100% oxygen while maintaining spontaneous respirations. If there is an IV in place, I would induce with lidocaine, glycopyrrolate, midazolam, and ketamine. In either case, I would have emergency airway equipment in the room and Ear, Nose, Throat (ENT) on standby for an emergency tracheostomy if the airway is lost.

Question 2

The surgeon plans to use carbon dioxide laser to ablate the papillomas. Would you intubate the patient? What are some potential problems with intubation for this case?

Answer 2

I would not intubate unless needed, as spontaneous ventilation without intubation allows the surgeon to work without interruption and it is preferred to laser-safe endotracheal tubes (ETTs). Some of the problems with intubation include airway bleeding, airway fire, obstruction of the surgical field, seeding of the papillomas into the distal airways, failure to pass the ETT as a result of the airway obstruction, increased airway resistance (by using a smaller-diameter ETT), and further airway scarring from repeated airway manipulations and surgeries.

Question 3

Do you need any special safety precautions while using a carbon dioxide laser?

Answer 3

Flammable surgical drapes should be minimized and wet towels should cover the face, neck, and shoulders to absorb laser energy. The eyes of the patient should be protected with shields or moist gauze pads. Safety glasses should be worn by operating room (OR) personnel. To prevent combustion, the FIO_2 should be as low as possible and nitrous oxide must not be used. In addition, laser-safe ETTs should be used with a saline-filled cuff, a fire extinguisher should be present in the room as well as a smoke evacuator for the laser, and special masks should be worn by personnel to prevent the spread of virus upon vaporization.

Question 4

How would you maintain anesthesia, with total intravenous anesthesia (TIVA) or inhalational agents?

Answer 4

Given that the patient is not intubated and maintenance of anesthesia with inhalational agents would lead to OR volatile gas contamination and variable depths of anesthesia for the patient during the procedure, I would perform a TIVA technique using propofol infusion (200–300 mcg/kg/min), remifentanil infusion (0.1–0.25 μg/kg/min), and aerosolized lidocaine.

Question 5

During the procedure the patient's saturation decreases from 98% to 75%. How will you treat this?

Answer 5

I would mask ventilate the child with 100% oxygen and, if needed, have the surgeon intubate the patient until the saturation improves.

Question 6

The surgeon tells you that the vocal cords are closed. What will you do?

Answer 6

I would provide gentle positive mask ventilation with 100% oxygen, and ask the surgeon to apply more aerosolized lidocaine onto the vocal cords after a bolus of propofol is given to deepen the anesthetic. If this does not break the laryngospasm, I would give succinylcholine.

Question 7

The surgeon has placed an endotracheal tube. While you are ventilating the patient smoke is seen arising from the airway. What do you do?

Answer 7

I would be concerned that the ETT has ignited. I would call for help, stop the flow of oxygen, disconnect the ETT from the gas source, and immediately extubate, ensuring that the entire ETT has been removed. A chest radiograph and a bronchoscopy should be performed to determine the extent of injury.

C. Postoperative Management

Postoperative Treatment of Airway Fire

Question 1

The patient was stabilized after the airway fire and mild edema was seen on bronchoscopy. How will you manage the patient?

Answer 1

After resecuring the airway with a smaller-sized ETT, I would continue with conservative measures by monitoring and giving humidified oxygen, steroids, and racemic epinephrine.

Question 2

The damage was mild and you decide to take the patient awake to the recovery room. The recovery room nurse calls to tell you that the patient is desaturating with decreased breath sounds bilaterally. Pulse is 140 BPM and blood pressure is 70/40 mmHg. What is your differential diagnosis?

Answer 2

My differential diagnosis includes tracheal tear, pneumothorax, airway obstruction, and bronchospasm.

Question 3

What will you do?

Answer 3

I would manually ventilate the patient with 100% oxygen to assess compliance, auscultate for bilateral breath sounds, suction out the ETT, check the circuit for no kinks or occlusions, obtain a chest X-ray, and send an ABG. In the event that my investigation leads me to a surgical etiology (tracheal tear) I would notify the surgeon.

Postoperative Carbon Dioxide Laser Complications

Question 4

A chest radiograph shows bilateral pneumothoraces and subcutaneous emphysema. What is your most likely diagnosis? How do you respond?

Answer 4

This is most likely a tracheal tear. I would call for help and prepare to emergently go into the operating room. I would have the surgeon place chest tubes or I would needle decompress the pneumothoraces depending on patient stability. Next, I would have the otolaryngologist replace an ETT with bronchoscope guidance and prepare for a tracheal repair.

Suggested Readings

Gregory GA, Andropoulos DB, eds. *Gregory's Pediatric Anesthesia*. 5th ed. Hoboken, NJ: Wiley-Blackwell; 2012.

Hines RL, Marschall KE, eds. *Stoelting's Anesthesia and Co-Existing Disease*. 5th ed. Philadelphia, PA: Churchill Livingstone; 2008.

Kadish H. Thoracic trauma. In: Fleisher GR, Ludwig S, Henretig FM, eds. *Textbook of Pediatric Emergency Medicine*. 5th ed. Philadelphia, PA: Lippincott, Williams & Wilkins; 2006:1433.

4 General: The Asthmatic Patient

Sana Na Javeed and Anna Kogan

A 57-year-old female is scheduled for an urgent laparoscopic, possibly open, cholecystectomy.

Past medical history: The patient has poorly controlled type 2 diabetes mellitus, well-controlled hypertension, and asthma, for which she was in the emergency room (ER) overnight for an exacerbation.

Physical exam: Pulse 66 bpm, BP 140/70 mmHg, RR 14, T 36.6°C, 96% on room air. Weight: 82 kg; height: 5'6". On physical exam, there is good neck extension and mouth opening, normal S1 and S2, mild expiratory wheeze.

EKG: Normal sinus rhythm.

Labs: Serum glucose is 165 mg/dL, normal chemistry and CBC.

Medications: Hydrochlorothiazide, metoprolol, albuterol metered-dose inhaler (MDI) prn, fluticasone MDI (Advair), montelukast (Singulair), and metformin.

A. Preoperative Evaluation

Question 1

Is this patient optimized for proposed urgent surgery? How do you know?

Answer 1

No, she is not. Based on the information given, this patient has poorly controlled asthma, as evidenced by her recent ER visit and also her pulmonary exam, which shows wheezing. Because this is an urgent case, we can delay surgery to administer inhalers or other medications, but rescheduling is not an option. Thus, I would want to give this patient her inhaler and see if this improves her wheezing before taking her to the OR. I would also obtain a baseline chest X-ray to rule out any infectious process, such as a pneumonia, that may be worsening her pulmonary status.

Question 2

Would you get a room air ABG?

Answer 2

Obtaining ABG results would not change management of this patient. My goal would be to treat her wheezing and avoid intraoperative episodes of bronchospasm. Thus I would not necessarily get a room air ABG because she seems to have acceptable oxygen saturation (>92%) on room air.

Question 3

Would you get flow-volume loops?

Answer 3

No, I would not. Obtaining pulmonary function tests (PFTs) would not provide me with any additional information beyond that from a thorough history and physical exam.

Question 4

You decide nonetheless to obtain a room air ABG. What do you expect it to show?

Answer 4

It depends on the state of her asthma. During initial asthma exacerbation, she would likely be hyperventilating to allow for increased air entry. In such a scenario, I would expect the patient to show a respiratory alkalosis secondary to decreased PCO_2 from the hyperventilation. However, if her asthma has progressed further, she would be tiring out with the use of accessory muscles for breathing, thereby retaining CO_2 and developing a respiratory acidosis. Assuming her wheezing doesn't represent an exacerbation, I would expect her ABG to be within normal range.

Question 5

You conclude that the patient is optimized even with current wheezing. Are you going to administer any medications before going to the OR?

Answer 5

Yes, I would administer an albuterol nebulizer, which is a β_2-receptor agonist resulting in airway smooth muscle relaxation and bronchodilation. The onset of action usually occurs within 5 minutes with peak effect in 1 hour and duration of action 4–6 hours. Ipratropium is an anticholinergic agent that blocks the muscarinic receptors of acetylcholine that are responsible for vagus nerve–mediated bronchoconstriction. I would also administer a dose of steroids as soon as possible. The peak effect will be in about 60 minutes.

Question 6

What is HbA1C?

Answer 6

HbA1C reflects the averages of a person's blood glucose levels over the past 3 months. The higher the level of glucose in the blood, the more glycated hemoglobin is formed. This test can be used to screen for and diagnose diabetes and to assess average daily glucose levels in diabetics over the past 3 months.

Question 7

Would you consider placing an epidural preoperatively in this patient? If so, at what level? Why?

Answer 7

Epidural anesthesia can be a great option for postoperative pain control for this patient, especially if there is a high chance of open surgery. It can be used intraoperatively to minimize opioid administration as well as postoperatively, which allows the patient to decrease splinting. I would not typically place an epidural on every cholecystectomy patient, however, unless there is a high chance of converting to an open procedure. I would place it at the level of about T8–T9.

B. Intraoperative Evaluation

Question 1

How would you induce anesthesia in this patient?

Answer 1

After preoxygenation with 100% oxygen, assuming a normal airway, I would conduct a slow, controlled induction using fentanyl, lidocaine, small doses of ketamine, propofol, and, after ensuring ventilation, rocuronium.

Question 2

Shortly after intubation, you notice the patient's $EtCO_2$ plummets to 10 mmHg, and there are high peak pressures. What is your differential diagnosis?

Answer 2

My differential would be bronchospasm, anaphylaxis, kinked endotracheal tube, mucus plug, and tension pneumothorax.

Question 3

Let's say this was bronchospasm. How would you treat this?

Answer 3

In the case of acute intraoperative bronchospasm, I would put the patient on 100% O_2 and manually bag ventilate her to directly assess compliance. If it is possible to ventilate the patient I would increase the inhalational agent concentration, administer albuterol, give benadryl (bronchospasm is secondary to an allergic reaction), and administer steroids (if not given already). If bronchospasm remains refractory, epinephrine would be administered in small doses starting with 10 mcg and doubling as needed.

Question 4

Is there a role for benadryl? Why or why not? How does it work?

Answer 4

Benadryl works as a histamine H1-receptor antagonist of effector cells in the respiratory tract, blood vessels, and GI smooth muscle. Although H1 blockers prevent a bronchoconstrictive response to histamine, they are ineffective in treating bronchial asthma, which is primarily due to other mediators. However, since it is unclear what triggered bronchospasm in this patient who is already predisposed to bronchospasm, I would administer benadryl.

Question 5

You can ventilate the patient. What ventilatory mode is the best for this patient? Why? What is the difference between peak and plateau pressures? Will both be elevated in an asthmatic patient?

Answer 5

In selecting a ventilator mode, attention needs to be given to providing adequately long expiratory time to avoid buildup of intrinsic or auto–positive end-expiratory pressure (PEEP). This can be facilitated by using smaller tidal volumes or higher inspiratory flow rates. I would consider changing the inspiratory/expiratory (I:E) ratio to 1:2.5 to give more time for expiration. I would use controlled ventilation for this patient, either pressure or volume controlled.

Question 6

What is meant by the terms *peak inspiratory pressure* and *plateau pressure*? How does asthma affect these indices?

Answer 6

Peak inspiratory pressure is the highest circuit pressure generated during an inspiratory cycle, providing an indication of dynamic compliance. Plateau pressure is the pressure measured during inspiratory pause (a time of no gas flow), indicating static compliance. In an asthmatic patient, with increased airway resistance due to bronchospasm, the peak inspiratory pressure will be increased, whereas plateau pressure will remain unchanged.

Question 7

The case goes uneventfully and the specimen is out. Vital signs are BP 156/84 mmHg, HR 92 bpm, O_2 saturation 94%. You suddenly notice ST depression in leads II, III, and aVF. What does this mean?

Answer 7

If I noticed ST depression in leads II, III, and aVF, I would be concerned about inferior wall ischemia.

Question 8

What would you do?

Answer 8

I would increase FiO_2 to 100% and ensure adequate oxygenation and ventilation. I would administer a short-acting beta blocker, such as esmolol, to decrease the heart rate, thereby decreasing myocardial O_2 demand, and ensure enough end diastolic pressures to allow for stable myocardial perfusion pressures. If there was significant blood loss I would give packed red blood cells (PRBC) to optimize oxygen carrying capacity.

Question 9

Would you administer nitroglycerin?

Answer 9

If the patient remains hemodynamically stable and the blood pressure is adequate, I would start a small dose of nitroglycerin because this drug is a potent coronary vasodilator. However, if the blood pressure is low, I would not start it.

C. Postoperative Evaluation

Question 1

ST changes have resolved and you have decided to extubate the patient in the PACU. What are your extubation criteria for this patient?

Answer 1

I would consider deep extubation if there is adequate tidal volume with minimal pressure support, especially if intubation was easy. If deep extubation is not possible, I would extubate the patient fully reversed, awake, following commands with good respiratory effort. My extubation criteria would be the same as for a nonasthmatic patient. Lidocaine as a bolus 1.5–2 mg/kg may help obtund airway reflexes during emergence.

Question 2

The patient complains of numbness in the fourth and fifth fingers. What do you think is the most likely cause?

Answer 2

Most likely this is from positioning of the arms during surgery and compression of the ulnar nerve at medial epicondyle.

Question 3

What would you do to address this?

Answer 3

I would tell the patient that this is most likely going to resolve on its own. However, if the numbness persists beyond 2 weeks, I would have the patient return to me for a visit. At that time I would do electromyographic (EMG) studies and order a neurology consult.

Question 4

The patient's glucose is 290 mg/dL. Would you treat this?

Answer 4

Yes, since high glucose levels increase risks of postoperative infection.

Question 5

What is the difference between NPH and regular insulin?

Answer 5

Regular human insulin is short- and fast-acting insulin and can easily be used in the perioperative setting as it can be given IV, with an onset within 15 minutes. NPH is intermediate-acting insulin given subcutaneously and is not typically used in the perioperative setting, especially since the patient is expected to be NPO for some time.

Question 6

Would you administer it subcutaneously or intramuscularly? Why?

Answer 6

I would use neither of these routes. My preference would be to administer IV insulin. Insulin can be given intravenously since subcutaneous or intramuscular (IM) administration depends on tissue blood flow and thus penetration can be unpredictable during surgery and immediately postoperatively.

Question 7

How does insulin work?

Answer 7

Most of the glucose absorbed following a meal is normally stored as glycogen, which only the liver and muscle are able to store in significant amounts. Insulin enhances glycogen synthesis and promotes uptake of glucose.

Question 8

Would you administer metformin? Why or why not?

Answer 8

I would not give metformin in this scenario because of its prolonged time of 7–8 hours to reach maximum plasma metformin concentrations for the drug to achieve its therapeutic benefit. It is also unclear if the patient will be on a diet by the time of its peak affect.

Suggested Readings

Butterworth JF. Respiratory physiology and anesthesia. In: Butterworth JF, Mackey DC, Wasnick JD, Morgan GE, Mikhail MS, eds. *Morgan & Mikhail's Clinical Anesthesiology*. 5th ed. New York: McGraw-Hill; 2013:487–526.

5 General: Liver Transplantation

Frederico Osorio

Stem 1

A 57-year-old, 72 kg male is scheduled for a liver transplant.

History of present illness: The patient suffers from chronic hepatic cirrhosis.

Patient medical history: hypertension (HTN), hypercholesterolemia.

Medications: He is currently on spironolactone, propranolol, metronidazole, and lactulose.

Physical exam: Vital signs: BP 126/80 mmHg, pulse 104 bpm, RR 28, oxygen 92% on RA. Mallampati score is 2 with a full range of motion. Dentition is normal. Auscultation reveals a systolic murmur due to a systolic anterior motion (SAM) of the mitral valve. There is a fluid-filled abdomen on exam. The rest of the exam is unremarkable.

Labs: Hb = 11.3 g/dL, white blood cell count (WBC) 11,000, Na = 132 mEq/L, K = 4.0 mEq/L.

A. Preoperative Evaluation

Cardiac

Question 1

How would you evaluate this patient's cardiac status?

Answer 1

First, a complete medical history and physical examination should be performed. From the history, I would want to know if he has had any episodes of chest pain, shortness of breath, or lightheadedness. I would also inquire about his baseline exercise tolerance by determining how many stairs he can climb comfortably. From the physical, I would listen to the heart sounds and assess for signs of congestive heart failure, such as jugular venous distention (JVD), pedal edema, and pulmonary edema, while keeping in mind that fluid overload can also be seen in cirrhosis. Finally, I would look at studies, specifically an EKG, and an echocardiogram because these patients are at high risk for pulmonary hypertension. If available, I would want to know the results of a stress test.

Liver Function Status

Question 2

How does this patient's history of cirrhosis affect your anesthetic management?

Answer 2

I would ensure the patient has large-bore PIV access, a preinduction arterial line, and a central line to allow adequate fluid resuscitation. In terms of induction, this patient most likely has ascites and so must be considered to have a full stomach. Since he could be volume depleted, it would be prudent to use cardiac stable agents for the induction. Higher than normal minimum alveolar concentration (MAC) values may be needed for maintenance because patients with cirrhosis often have a history of alcoholism. Finally, I would avoid using drugs that undergo significant hepatic metabolism.

Question 3

What are the factors associated with liver disease that lead to the accumulation of ascites?

Answer 3

The factors that lead to ascites are hypoalbuminemia, portal hypertension, and water retention (secondary to secretion of antinatriuretic factors and antidiuretic hormone [ADH]).

Question 4

What is hepatorenal syndrome?

Answer 4

Hepatorenal syndrome is an often fatal condition that is associated with rapid functional renal failure secondary to fulminate liver disease and cirrhosis.

Question 5

Your resident informs you that there is no recent echocardiogram on file. Would you delay the case?

Answer 5

Yes, I would delay it because I want to fully understand the severity and symptomology associated with the systolic murmur, because this would affect my anesthetic management. I also want to know if this patient has pulmonary HTN, because severe pulmonary HTN (>50 mmHg) is a contraindication to a transplant.

B. Intraoperative Management

Monitors

Question 1

What kind of monitoring devices would you use in this patient?

Answer 1

In addition to the standard ASA monitors (pulse oximeter, noninvasive blood pressure [NIBP], EKG, $EtCO_2$, and temperature) I would place an arterial line, a central line catheter (large 12 Fr), and transesophageal echocardiography (TEE).

Question 2

Do you have any concerns about the use of TEE in this particular patient?

Answer 2

Yes. The use of TEE may cause rupture and bleeding of esophageal varices. However, if extreme caution is exercised during the insertion and manipulation of the TEE probe, the likelihood of this complication has been found to be very low. In this case with the history of SAM and the high hemodynamic variations expected on a liver transplant procedure, I consider the use of TEE to be essential.

Hematological Considerations

Question 3

Assuming the patient is medically optimized, would you perform an intrathecal morphine injection for perioperative pain control in this patient?

Answer 3

No. Liver dysfunction is associated with multiple coagulation derangements (prolonged prothrombin time [PT], elevated international normalized ratio [INR], thrombocytopenia, platelet dysfunction). Regional anesthesia is an unacceptable high-risk procedure for this patient.

Question 4

Which blood products, if any, would you want in the room?

Answer 4

Because these procedures are associated with massive blood loss and coagulopathy, I would want at least 10 units of PRBC, 5–10 units of fresh frozen plasma (FFP), 100 units of platelets, and 10 units of cryoprecipitate.

Induction

Question 5

How would you induce this patient?

Answer 5

Because this patient likely has increased intra-abdominal pressure from ascites, I would treat him as I would for a full stomach. Thus, I would premedicate with sodium citrate, metoclopramide, and an H2 antagonist. Then, I would place the patient in reverse Trendelenburg position to reduce the risk of any passive regurgitation. Assuming a normal airway, I would perform a rapid sequence induction (RSI) with cricoid pressure using etomidate, and succinylcholine after adequate prehydration and placement of a preinduction arterial line.

Question 6

Immediately after induction, the BP rapidly decreases to 75/40 mmHg, and HR is 80 bpm. What are you going to do?

Answer 6

I would immediately place the patient on 100% oxygen, look at the monitors to rule out a malignant arrhythmia, and pulse oximeter to rule out hypoxia, hypercarbia while feeling for a carotid pulse. Assuming all of these parameters were normal, I would open the fluids and administer a low dose of phenylephrine to improve the BP.

Preanhepatic Phase

Question 7

What are the stages of a liver transplant surgery?

Answer 7

1. Preanhepatic phase: Period when the native liver is mobilized and dissected
2. Anhepatic phase: Period when the native liver is removed
3. Reperfusion phase: Period during which the new donor liver is anastomosed

Question 8

Shortly after the surgeon has made the incision, you notice a very active suctioning sound. The patient starts turning gradually hypotensive although no significant blood loss has occurred. How would you assess this? What is your differential diagnosis? How would you manage the patient?

Answer 8

I would immediately look at the vitals and ensure the patient is not hypoxic, hypo- or hypercarbic, or in a malignant rhythm. Assuming all of these were normal, the most common initial cause of hypotension at the early stages of liver transplantation is hypovolemia due to the combination of the vasodilatory effects of the induction agents and the drainage of ascites. Thus, I would administer a bolus of a colloid-containing solution and continue giving boluses according to the central venous pressure (CVP) values and the appearance of the heart cavities on the TEE.

Anhepatic Stage

Question 9

Twenty-five minutes into the anhepatic phase you notice a sustained period of hypotension, with no significant increases in blood loss. CVP = 11 mmHg, hemoglobin/hematocrit (H/H) = 10 g/dL/L, 30%. How would you evaluate this situation?

Answer 9

First, I would look at the patient's other vitals to make sure they are stable. During the anhepatic stage, blood loss is not the typical cause of hypotension, especially after having a normal CVP value. After ruling out a mechanical cause of the problem by looking over the surgical field and asking the surgical team to check for sponges and evaluating suction containers, I would focus on contractility issues. First, I would review the electrocardiogram tracing, looking for prolongation of the QT interval (hypocalcemia) and ST interval (changes during acute ischemic events). I would also look at the trans esophageal echocardiogram (TEE) to evaluate for regional wall motion abnormalities +/-, global hypokinesia.

Question 10

What is the difference between the "traditional technique" and the "piggyback" technique during the anhepatic phase? How do they affect your anesthetic management?

Answer 10

In the traditional technique, the surgeon performs a complete vascular occlusion by clamping the inferior vena cava (IVC), suprahepatic vena cava, hepatic artery, and the portal vein. As a result, venous return decreases by 50–60% and severe hypotension with a compensatory tachycardia may occur from the low CO. To prevent this, veno-venous bypass (VVBP) would have to be initiated and the complications associated with VVBP, such as arm edema, air embolism, and vascular injury, would have to be treated. The alternative is for me to volume load the patient with a target CVP of 10–20 mmHg and administer vasopressor boluses prior to clamping of the vessels. In the piggyback technique, the vena cava is partially occluded, making the surgery more challenging but eliminating the need for VVBP or the hemodynamic fluctuations encountered with the traditional technique.

Reperfusion Stage

Question 11

The surgeon notifies you that he or she is about to "reperfuse." How would you prepare for this?

Answer 11

Reperfusing the transplanted liver is one of the most critical moments of the operation, because the recipient's blood will flush through the new liver and force multiple metabolic products into the main circulation. This will lead to a decrease in cardiac contractility, CO, systemic vascular resistance (SVR), and abrupt rises in pulmonary vascular resistance and serum hydrogen and potassium ion concentrations.

I would prepare by keeping the patient's intravascular volume optimized, checking the ABG and H/H to correct any acid–base electrolyte disorder, and transfuse according to hemodynamic and H/H levels. I would have pressors, calcium, insulin, sodium bicarbonate, and blood products in line ready for use. Once the patient's status was optimized, I would notify the surgeon to start the reperfusion process.

Question 12

What is meant by the "reperfusion syndrome?"

Answer 12

Reperfusion syndrome is hemodynamic instability, of unknown mechanism usually occurring during the first 5 minutes of reperfusion, that is associated with hyperkalemia and hemodynamic fluctuations such as hypotension, bradycardia, elevated pulmonary artery pressure (PAP), and supraventricular tachycardia.

C. Postoperative Care

Postoperative Bleeding

Question 1

You are paged to the surgical intensive care unit (SICU) because the nurse has just noticed that the drains from the abdominal cavity have been filling up rapidly. What should you do at this point?

Answer 1

I would immediately go to the patient's bedside and evaluate his vital signs to make sure they are stable while asking the nurse to notify the surgeon. I would send for an ABG, H&H, and thromboelastography (TEG) samples. If hypotension was present I would give a bolus of 500 mL of lactated Ringer's (LR) immediately, as well as a dose of phenylephrine to recover the BP.

Coagulopathy and Anemia

Question 2

While you are administering the first bolus of fluids, the laboratory calls to inform you that the TEG maximum amplitude (MA) value is below the normal values. An ABG shows: Hb = 9.2 g/dL, pH = 7.32, $PaCO_2$ = 53 mmHg, BE = −2. CVP = 4 cm H_2O, BP = 98/54 mmHg. What would you do?

Answer 2

The low MA value suggests to me an issue related to the platelet component. Thus, I would start transfusing two bags of platelets, watching closely the CVP value since a high CVP may lead to congestion of the new liver and trigger further bleeding and/or graft dysfunction. The other results suggest anemia, which can be worsened by the transfusion of non-red blood cells containing fluids. Therefore, I would prepare the patient for blood transfusion, making sure of the availability of five units of blood. The ABG result suggests the presence of mild respiratory acidosis, so I would adjust the mechanical ventilation by increasing the respiratory rate or tidal volume as tolerated.

Question 3

After the transfusion of two units of platelets the patient's nurse calls you to tell you the patient's bleeding had initially improved but is now worsening again. How do you respond?

Answer 3

I would immediately evaluate the patient at the bedside. I will check vital signs to verify stability. Based on the clinical presentation of recurring hemorrhage and the findings from the TEG results, the diagnosis of fibrinolysis is more clear. At this point, I would order a dose of intravenous aminocaproic acid and check the level of fibrinogen to determine if a transfusion of cryoprecipitate is required.

Suggested Readings

Hines RL, Marschall KE, eds. *Stoelting's Anesthesia and Coexisting Disease*. 5th ed. Philadelphia, PA: Saunders Elsevier; 2008.

O'Riordan J, O'Beirne HA, Young Y, Bellamy MC. Effects of desflurane and isoflurane on splanchnic microcirculation during major surgery. *Br J Anaesth*. 1997;78(1):95–96.

Prasad S, Dhiman RK, Duseja A, Chawla YK, Sharma A, Agarwal R. Lactulose improves cognitive functions and health-related quality of life in patients with cirrhosis who have minimal hepatic encephalopathy. *Hepatology*. 45(3):549–559.

Randolph H, Steadman MD. Anesthesia for liver transplant surgery. *Anesthesiol Clin North Am*. 2004; 22:687–711.

6 General: Renal Transplantation

Ruchir Gupta, Sheryl Glassman, and Anita Gupta

Stem 2

A 55-year-old female is scheduled for a cadaveric kidney transplant harvested 16 hours ago. She underwent dialysis 25 hours ago. She has a history of diabetes mellitus, hypertension, and coronary artery disease. Medications include glipizide, metoprolol, and alprazolam. Vital signs are HR 75, BP 180/90 mm Hg, RR 24, RA saturation 97%. Hb = 11.3 g/dL, platelets = 235 K, WBC = 10.1 K/mcL, Na = 140 mEq/L, K = 5.2 mEq/L.

A. Preoperative Evaluation

Evaluation

Question 1

What are the systemic manifestations of chronic renal failure?

Answer 1

Chronic renal failure has effects on multiple organ systems:

Cardiac—patients are at risk for hypertension (HTN), congestive heart failure (CHF), cardiomyopathy, coronary artery disease (CAD), and hyperdynamic circulation.

Pulmonary—patients may have pulmonary edema.

GI—gastroparesis, gastritis, and pancreatitis

Hematological—anemia, coagulopathy, metabolic acidosis, hyperkalemia, hyperphosphatemia, hypocalcemia, and hyperuricemia

Neurological—encephalopathy, peripheral neuropathy, seizures, myoclonus, and asterixis

Question 2

What hematological issues are you concerned about in this patient?

Answer 2

In addition to a baseline chronic anemia, I am concerned that this patient may have a coagulopathy because many patients with chronic renal failure (CRF) have thrombocytopathy and decreased prothrombin levels.

Question 3

Would you order any additional preoperative tests in this patient?

Answer 3

Yes. I would want an EKG, a chest radiograph, coagulation profile, and tests for liver function enzymes, bilirubin, and albumin.

Hyperkalemia

Question 4

Would you delay the case to correct this patient's serum potassium level?

Answer 4

No. Chronic hyperkalemia secondary to renal failure is an expected finding with this patient. As long as she was not symptomatic, I would not delay the case. I would have medications such as calcium, insulin, glucose, bicarbonate, and a beta agonist in the operating room before induction, however.

Question 5

What if the patient's repeat serum potassium comes back at 6.0 mEq/L? Would you delay the case then?

Answer 5

Yes. At 6.0 mEq/L the serum K^+ level is at a life-threatening level and can lead to ventricular fibrillation and asystole. I would delay the case and immediately begin treatment with calcium, insulin, bicarbonate, beta agonists, and glucose.

Question 6

The surgeon says that is a normal laboratory finding in a patient with renal failure and this is an emergency procedure. How would you respond?

Answer 6

I would inform the surgeon of two things:

1. Renal transplants are not emergent cases. Cadaveric kidneys can be maintained for 36–48 hours to optimize the patient, and preoperative optimization will ensure a better outcome for the patient.
2. While some patients with end-stage renal disease (ESRD) do suffer from chronic hyperkalemia, a value of 6.0 mEq/L can be lethal and thus cannot be considered a normal finding. At this level, the patient may develop a malignant cardiac rhythm at any time.

Medications

Question 7

The patient informs you that she did not take any of her medications this morning. How would you manage this patient's home medication regimen before bringing her to the operating room?

Answer 7

This patient is currently on glipizide for diabetes mellitus (DM), metoprolol for HTN, and alprazolam for presumed anxiety. I would hold her glipizide because oral hypoglycemics should not be administered since the patient will be NPO and hypoglycemia may result from its administration. Conversely, I would continue her metoprolol because any patient on long-term beta-blocker therapy should continue it to reduce the risk of morbidity and mortality during such procedures. Finally, I would ask the patient to take her normal dose alprazolam so that she doesn't have any symptoms of withdrawal or anxiety before arriving to the OR. Additionally, if she does appear anxious, I could titrate in a low dose of Midazolam before bringing her to the OR.

Premedication

Question 8

Would you administer any premedications to this patient?

Answer 8

It depends. If this patient appeared anxious, I would begin with verbal reassurance. If she continued to be anxious, I would consider administering a low dose of midazolam. Next, because this patient is at risk for gastroparesis, I would administer sodium citrate as well as promotility agents such as metoclopromide, which will promote gastric emptying.

B. Intraoperative Management

Regional vs. General Anesthesia Techniques

Question 1

Could you do this case under regional?

Answer 1

No. this patient likely has a coagulopathy secondary to uricemia leading to decreased von Willebrand factor (vWF) levels. Thus, I would want to avoid neuraxial techniques completely.

Monitors

Question 2

How would you monitor this patient?

Answer 2

I would place the standard ASA monitors, a neuromuscular blockade monitor, preinduction arterial line, and a central line to optimize intravascular volume and follow CVP trends.

Induction

Question 3

How would you induce this patient?

Answer 3

Assuming the patient has a reassuring airway, I would preoxygenate with 100% O_2 and perform rapid sequence induction with fentanyl, etomidate, and succinylcholine. I would perform rapid sequence induction technique to reduce the risk of aspiration in this patient, who likely has gastroparesis secondary to chronic renal insufficiency.

Maintenance

Question 4

Assuming you decided to do this case under general anesthesia, what agents would you use for maintenance?

Answer 4

I would use a balanced anesthetic technique with a volatile anesthetic, an opioid, and a muscle relaxant. In terms of inhalation agent, I would use Desflurane because it does not have nephrotoxic potential and has a rapid wash-in and washout time. I would avoid sevoflurane because its metabolism can produce nephrotoxic agents such as compound A and fluoride. Opioids can be used to maintain analgesia, although I would avoid meperidine and morphine because both depend on renal clearance and have active metabolites that can accumulate (morphine-3-glucuronide and morphine-6-glucuronide and normeperidine, respectively). Morphine-6-glucuronide accumulation can lead to worsening of respiratory depression. Normeperidine accumulation can lead to neurotoxic effects such as seizure activity. Finally, for neuromuscular blockade I would use cisatracurium since metabolism and elimination are independent of the renal pathway.

Preparation for Graft Attachment

Question 5

The surgeon informs you that he is about to clamp the iliac vessels. What medications would you administer at this time?

Answer 5

I would administer heparin before clamping (to prevent clotting) and have the surgeon inject verapamil or papaverine into the graft arteries before revascularization (to prevent arterial vasopasm) and mannitol/furosemide after graft reperfusion (to induce diuresis).

Renal Graft Reperfusion

Question 6

The kidney graft vessels and ureter are anastomosed and the clamp is now removed. The patient's blood pressure quickly plummets to 77/38 mmHg. How do you respond?

Answer 6

I would immediately check the patient's other vital signs, including heart rate, pulse, end-tidal CO_2, and oxygen saturation, and an EKG for any malignant arrhythmia. Hypotension immediately following unclamping is most likely due to the washout of vasoactive substances from the renal graft. Treatment would be primarily supportive. Thus, assuming all other vital signs were stable, I would open fluids wide, administer pressors such as phenylephrine or ephedrine, and send for an ABG with electrolytes.

Question 7

The EKG monitor shows peaked T waves. What is your response?

Answer 7

This is most likely due to hyperkalemia from the preservative fluid of the new kidney. Thus, I would administer calcium gluconate for myocardial protection and then administer insulin, glucose, bicarbonate, and a beta agonist to decrease the serum levels of K^+.

C. Postoperative Management

Extubation

Question 1

Would you extubate this patient?

Answer 1

It depends on the clinical course. If the patient demonstrated hemodynamic stability with stable vital signs, was awake and alert, followed commands, was pulling in adequate tidal volumes (>6 mL/kg), and was full reversed and the operation was devoid of large fluid shifts, I would extubate. However, if the patient developed some unforeseen intraoperative event or had massive fluid shifts and was not able to breathe on her own, I would prefer to leave the patient intubated overnight.

Postoperative Oliguria

Question 2

You are paged stat to the PACU for decreased urine output. What is your differential?

Answer 2

Oliguria can be categorized as prerenal, intrarenal, and postrenal. Prerenal oliguria is due to hypoperfusion, which is usually caused by hypovolemia. Thus, I would check input and outputs (I/Os) to assess how much fluid the patient has been given, check CVP readings if there is a central line, and send for electrolytes to assess for signs of dehydration such as hypernatremia. I would also look at her skin turgor and mucus membranes. Postrenal pathology is usually due to a kinked Foley catheter or bladder obstruction. Intrarenal oliguria is often due to the presence of nephrotoxic substances. A urinalysis with casts would be helpful in confirming the diagnosis. Additionally, this patient maybe experiencing graft rejection, toxic injury, or vessel occlusion.

Question 3

What are some laboratory differences between prerenal and renal oliguria?

Answer 3

Common indices to differentiate prerenal and renal oliguria include urine osmolality, urine sodium, fractional excretion of sodium (FENa), and urine:serum creatinine ratio. Urine osmolarity (mOsm/L) is greater than 500 in patients with prerenal etiology and less than 400 in patients with renal etiology. Urine sodium is less than 20 mEq/L in prerenal patients and greater than 40 mEq/L in patients with renal etiology. The urine:serum creatinine ratio is greater than 40 in prerenal etiology patients and less than 20 in patients with renal etiology. The blood urea nitrogen (BUN)/creatinine (Crt) ratio in prerenal etiology patients is greater than 20 and often less than 10–15 in renal etiology patients. FENa, measured as a percentage, is less than 1% in prerenal patients and greater than 2% in renal patients.

Nausea

Question 4

You are paged from the postoperative care unit because the patient is complaining of nausea. How will you respond?

Answer 4

Nausea here has several possible etiologies. My first response would be to rule out hypoxia, hypoventilation, and hypotension. I would also evaluate for anxiety, postoperative pain, and opioid side effect. Assuming all of this was normal, I would administer a dose of a 5-HT3 blocker, such as Zofran.

Suggested Readings

Barash PG, Cullen BF, Stoelting RK, Cahalan M, Stock CM, eds. *Clinical Anesthesia*. 6th ed. Philadelphia, PA: Lippincott Williams & Wilkins; 2009.

Miller RD, Eriksson LI, Fleisher LA, Wiener-Kornish JP, Young WL, eds. *Miller's Anesthesia*. 7th ed. Philadelphia, PA: Churchill Livingstone Elsevier; 2010.

Yao F, Fontes ML, Malhotra V, eds. *Yao and Artusio's Anesthesiology: Problem-Oriented Patient Management*. 7th ed. Philadelphia, PA: Lippincott Williams & Wilkins; 2011.

7 Endocrine: Thyroidectomy

Ruchir Gupta

Stem 1

A 35-year-old female with a weight of 55 kg is scheduled for resection of a goiter. The patient has had dysphagia and dyspnea for the past month.

Past medical history: asthma

Medications: albuterol, propylthiouracil

Allergies: no known drug allergies (NKDA)

Physical exam: Vital signs: HR 130 bpm, BP 180/95 mmHg, RR 20

Airway: Mallampati II, full cervical range of motion

Cardiovascular: tachycardic

Pulmonary: clear to auscultation

Labs: Hb 11.2 g/dL, platelets 280 K, Na 135 mEq/L

A. Preoperative Evaluation

Hemodynamics

Question 1

Is this patient ready for surgery?

Answer 1

No. This patient is displaying signs of thyrotoxicosis, most likely secondary to increased secretion of the thyroid hormone from the goiter. I would delay the case until this patient is medically managed and made euthyroid.

Question 2

The surgeon says this is an emergency case. How will you respond?

Answer 2

I would inform the surgeon that this is not an emergency case. Thyroidectomy is an elective procedure and this patient needs to be medically managed before taking her to the OR, to prevent life-threatening hemodynamic changes. Currently, this patient is receiving only propylthiouracil (PTU). I would substitute or add methimazole to her regimen for 6–8 weeks because PTU by itself is not accomplishing the goal. I would also want this patient to take potassium iodide for 10–14 days.

Beta Blockers

Question 3

Are beta blockers helpful in these types of patients? Would you use it in this particular patient?

Answer 3

Beta blockers do not affect the underlying thyroid pathology but are helpful in reducing the signs and symptoms of thyroid pathology such as hypertension and tachycardia. However, in this particular patient, I would want to only administer B1-selective agents such as metoprolol and avoid drugs that block B2 because of exacerbation of her asthma.

Optimization

Question 4

If this were a true surgical emergency, what steps would you take to prepare this patient for surgery?

Answer 4

I would take steps to reduce the possibility of developing a thyroid storm. I would administer antithyroid drugs such as methimazole and PTU to decrease thyroid hormone synthesis, iopanoic acid to reduce triiodothyronine (T3) levels, and glucocorticoids to block peripheral conversion of thyroxine (T4) to T3.

Airway

Question 5

The patient returns 2 months later with HR of 88 bpm, BP 110/70 mmHg, RR 12. How would you examine this patient's airway?

Answer 5

I would perform a focused history and physical. From the history, I would ask this patient about her dysphagia and dyspnea, assessing whether it has been getting worse or is stable, are there any exacerbating or alleviating factors, or have there been any prior intubations and if she had these symptoms at the time. From the physical, I would perform an external airway exam to assess if there is any neck compression by the goiter. I would also perform an internal exam to see if there is any gross deviation in the oropharynx. Most importantly, I would want a flow-volume loop test to assess if there is any intra- or extrathoracic compression and also look at any CT scans that might help me quantify the size and extent of the tumor.

Antithyroid Therapy

Question 6

Would you continue this patient's antithyroid medicines the morning of surgery or would you ask that they be discontinued before surgery?

Answer 6

All antithyroid medications should be continued until the morning of surgery.

B. Intraoperative Management

Monitoring

Question 1

Does this patient need a pulmonary artery (PA) catheter for the case?

Answer 1

Based on the information given, I do not think this patient needs a PA catheter at this time because I can monitor her hemodynamic status accurately with standard ASA monitors as well as with a central line and an arterial line (A-line), if necessary. A PA catheter increases this patient's risk of infection, pneumothorax, vascular and cardiac injury, and bleeding. Thus, in this case I do not believe the benefits outweigh the risks.

Question 2

Would you place an A-line? Why?

Answer 2

Yes. In this patient I would want an A-line, which I could use for beat-to-beat monitoring of the blood pressure at critical times during the induced hypotension period, serial ABGs, and H/H assessments.

Airway

Question 3

How would you secure the airway?

Answer 3

Given the patient's history of dysphagia and dyspnea and presumed airway mass effect from the goiter, I would perform an awake fiber-optic intubation (AFOI).

Anesthesia

Question 4

Your resident suggests using ketamine to keep the patient spontaneously breathing during the FOI. How do you respond?

Answer 4

Yes, only if the patient cannot tolerate an AFOI technique despite adequate airway topicalization with nebulized lidocaine and Cetacaine spray and she remains euthyroid on the day of surgery, since ketamine can raise her blood pressure and heart rate.

Bleeding

Question 5

Does this patient need a higher MAC for anesthetic maintenance?

Answer 5

No. MAC values are the same for a euthyroid patient as for a hyperthyroid patient.

Question 6

Midway through the case, the surgeon informs you that he accidentally cut into an artery and the patient is losing massive amounts of blood. The patient's BP now reads 85/70 mmHg. What do you do?

Answer 6

I would immediately place the patient on 100% oxygen and look at other vital signs and make sure the patient is not hypoxic, hypercarbic, or in a malignant arrhythmia. Next, I would open fluids wide while drawing a stat ABG to determine an H/H. I would also call for blood and administer a direct-acting agent such as phenylephrine as a temporizing measure.

Question 7

Can you use ephedrine as a temporizing measure?

Answer 7

Yes, but only if the patient is made euthyroid. Hyperthyroid patients may have an exaggerated response to indirect agents.

C. Postoperative Care

Extubation

Question 1

Would you extubate this patient?

Answer 1

It depends. If the case went uneventfully and the patient was fully reversed, following commands, and taking adequate tidal volumes, I would extubate. If, however, this was a complicated case with massive transfusion requirements and swelling at the surgical site and the patient was not able to take adequate tidal volumes, I would leave the patient intubated and sedated overnight.

Postoperative Stridor

Question 2

You are paged from the PACU because the patient has developed stridor. What is your differential?

Answer 2

My differential diagnosis is recurrent laryngeal nerve injury, laryngospasm, tracheomalacia, hematoma formation at the surgical site, inadequate muscle relaxant reversal, and residual anesthetic.

Question 3

How would you determine if the cause of the injury was bilateral recurrent laryngeal nerve (RLN) damage?

Answer 3

To assess for bilateral RLN injury, I would ask the patient to say "EE." In bilateral injury, the patient would be aphonic.

Question 4

A stat electrolyte panel reveals a low serum calcium level. What do you think could have caused this?

Answer 4

Inadvertent removal of the parathyroid glands can result in hypocalcemia with resulting respiratory distress. Usually this does not manifest until 24 hours postoperatively.

Question 5

What is Chvostek's sign?

Answer 5

Chvostek's sign is facial nerve excitability due usually to hypocalcemia.

Suggested Readings

Atchabahian A, Gupta R, eds. *The Anesthesia Guide*. New York: McGraw-Hill; 2013.

Hines RL, Marschall KE, eds. *Stoelting's Anesthesia and Co-Existing Disease*. 5th ed. Philadelphia, PA: Saunders; 2008.

8 Endocrine: Carcinoid Tumor

Dieman La and Minh Chau Joe Tran

Stem 2

A 50-year-old, 90 kg female is scheduled for resection of an abdominal carcinoid tumor. She has a medical history of chronic obstructive pulmonary disease (COPD) from chronic smoking, hypertension, hyperlipidemia, and a decreased activity level. Medications include hydrochlorothiazide (HCTZ), lisinopril, and simvastatin. She was diagnosed with the carcinoid tumor with hepatic metastasis 3 months ago. Vital signs are BP 118/77 mmHg, HR 76 bpm, RR 14, O_2 saturation 97% on RA. Labs: Na 138 mEq/L, K 3.2 mEql/L, Hb 12.2 g/dL.

A. Preoperative Evaluation

Carcinoid Tumor

Question 1

How would you evaluate this patient's carcinoid tumor?

Answer 1

First, I would determine if the tumor is functional or nonfunctional through a focused history and physical. Functional tumors secrete bioactive substances causing a wide sequelae of symptoms including classic carcinoid signs of flushing, diarrhea, and labile blood pressures. Thus, from the history, I would ask if the patient has experienced any bronchospasm, diarrhea, dramatic swings in BP, or any increased heart rate or palpitations (supraventricular tachycardia [SVT]).
From the physical, I would examine the patient for any carcinoid signs:

General: Is the patient alert? Does the patient appear inappropriately drowsy? Increased daytime somnolence is one of the lesser known effects of elevated serotonin.

From a cardiac standpoint, is the heart rate normal? Are there any heart murmurs (carcinoid tumors are associated with right heart lesions)?

Respiratory: Are there any signs of wheezing?

GI: Is there an enlarged liver? Abdominal pain?

Lastly, I would look at any imaging studies to see where the tumor is located and to determine its overall size. I would see if there are any labs in regard to

5-hydroxyindoleacetic acid (5-HIAA) levels, for diagnostic and monitoring purposes.

Question 2

Do you expect this patient's carcinoid to be functional?

Answer 2

Since only 25% of tumors produce mediators, most patients do not have functional tumors. Tumors that are considered nonfunctional produce vague symptoms through mass effect and can present as abdominal pain, GI bleed, and bowel obstruction.

Even still, patients with functional intestinal carcinoid tumors generally do not have symptoms because the vasoactive substances are cleared by the portal circulation and metabolized by the liver. Mediator-producing tumors that are not part of the portal circulation, such as bronchial, ovarian, and hepatic tumors, have a tendency to produce more symptoms. Given that this patient has hepatic metastasis, there is a high likelihood that the tumor is functional.

Question 3

How is a carcinoid tumor diagnosed and should it be monitored?

Answer 3

Most carcinoid tumors are found incidentally during surgeries for other reasons. Assuming this patient is symptomatic, the tumor can be confirmed with urinary 5-HIAA and serum levels of chromogranin A. The gold standard for locating functional tissue is still radiolabeled somatostatin analog scintigraphy, such as radiolabeled octreotide. Although not necessary, monitoring urinary 5-HIAA levels will help assess the disease progression and may help intraoperative management of the patient.

Cardiac

Question 4

How would you evaluate the patient's cardiac status preoperatively?

Answer 4

Again, I would start with a detailed history and physical. From the history, I would want to quantify this patient's decreased baseline activity level. Also, any recent episodes of chest pain or shortness of breath should be elicited.

From the physical, I would want to know if this patient has heart murmurs or signs of CHF—specifically signs of right heart failure such as JVD or pedal edema, since these patients are at risk for right-sided valvular lesions.

Question 5

What type of cardiac testing would you order?

Answer 5

I would order an echocardiogram to evaluate if there are any carcinoid-related valvular issues. A stress echo is preferred given the patient's decreased baseline functionality. I would also obtain a baseline EKG.

Question 6

What structural changes would you expect to find on an echocardiogram?

Answer 6

Tricuspid regurgitation is the most frequent phenomenon. Tricuspid stenosis may occur also. Pulmonary insufficiency or stenosis has been reported as well. All of these could lead to right-side heart failure.

Pulmonary

Question 7

How would you evaluate this patient's pulmonary function?

Answer 7

First, I would obtain a detailed history and physical.

From the history, I would assess whether the patient had any increased incidences of bronchospasm, any dyspnea with exercise, and any increased oxygen requirement concerning for metabolite release vs. carcinoid-associated right heart failure.

From the physical, I would also auscultate for wheezing, rhonchi, or rales. I would observe to see if the patient has any increased work of breathing.

Question 8

Would you obtain PFTs?

Answer 8

No. PFTs have not been shown to affect anesthetic management in most cases (unless, of course, resection involves the respiratory system). For this patient, I can obtain most of my information from a detailed history and physical and, if necessary, a chest X-ray at most.

Metabolic

Question 9

What substances are released by a carcinoid tumor?

Answer 9

Carcinoid tumors are derived from enterochromaffin cells. They may release an array of mediators, including serotonin, histamine, catecholamines, tachykinin, bradykinin, prostaglandin, and vasoactive intestinal peptide. The substances can cause flushing, diarrhea, abdominal pain, bronchospasm, palpitation, hypertension or hypotension, and heart failure. The serotonin metabolite 5-HIAA collected in a 24-hour urine sample can be used to diagnose and monitor tumor activity.

Question 10

What other labs would you obtain for this patient other than the ones previously mentioned?

Answer 10

As for any major surgery, I would make sure to obtain CBC, electrolytes, and coagulopathy studies (PTT, PT/INR). I would make sure her electrolytes are within normal limits and are not indicative of chronic diarrhea or dehydration.

I would also order crossmatched blood for this patient, especially since there are lesions in the liver.

Question 11

What are your anesthetic concerns for a patient with a carcinoid tumor?

Answer 11

In addition to the routine cardiac and pulmonary precautions, I am concerned about the precipitation of a carcinoid crisis. Thus, I would ask the patient if there are specific triggers for her carcinoid tumor. Stress, anxiety, exercise, or certain foods high in serotonin such as coffee, cheese, alcohol, and bananas are known triggers for carcinoid symptoms.

I would be sure to reduce preoperative anxiety, as well as stress from the intubation, surgery, or pain, as all of these factors can precipitate hormone release. Finally, I would also be vigilant about direct surgical tumor manipulation since that can trigger a carcinoid crisis.

Question 12

What would you advise in regard to the patient's medications?

Answer 12

Although no specific guidelines exist, like for any major surgery I would advise the patient to stop taking her lisinopril, as this may worsen the large blood pressure variance observed during induction. Her antihypertensive regimen may also make her hypotension refractory and the HCTZ may worsen her volume status.

Most importantly, given the fact that she has metastasis to the liver, she may have increased circulating metabolites. One of the main goals of perioperative management of carcinoid tumors is to control tumor activity. This can be achieved by octreotide prior to surgery. Octreotide is similar to somatostatin in that it inhibits serotonin, vasoactive intestinal peptide, histamine, and a wide variety of other hormones. An octreotide infusion can be started before surgery, and small boluses can be given when signs of vasoactive hormone release are observed intraoperatively.

B. Intraoperative Management

Monitoring

Question 1

What kind of monitors and or equipment would you require for this patient?

Answer 1

In addition to the standard ASA monitors, I would like to have a preinduction A-line to provide better vigilance of hemodynamic variables. I would also want a central line to have adequate IV access as well as to volume resuscitate during a carcinoid crisis. I would like to have anesthesia depth monitoring, such as a bispectral index (BIS) monitor, so that I can titrate to provide an adequate level of sedation while avoiding over-anesthetizing.

Question 2

What is the effect of carcinoid tumor on MAC value?

Answer 2

An increased serotonin level will result in lower MAC value and delayed awakening. The higher the serotonin level, the lower the MAC value.

Induction

Question 3

How would you induce this patient?

Answer 3

My goal is to maintain hemodynamic stability and reduce the risk of carcinoid crisis by avoiding hypotension, catecholamine secretion, and histamine release. Thus, assuming a normal airway, I would perform a slow, controlled induction with fentanyl, etomidate, and rocuronium.

Question 4

Are there any drugs you would avoid using during induction in this patient?

Answer 4

I would avoid use of the following neuromuscular blockers:

- Atracurium, because it is associated with histamine release and potentiates the carcinoid crisis
- Succinylcholine, because the fasciculations could cause an increase in intra-abdominal pressures, thus inadvertently causing tumor manipulation.

Maintenance

Question 5

How would you maintain anesthesia for the patient?

Answer 5

I would use a balanced technique using oxygen/air, isoflurane/sevoflurane, fentanyl, and rocuronium.

Question 6

What type of pain medication would you or would you not offer this patient?

Answer 6

I would not offer this patient any morphine, as this, too, can cause histamine release. Otherwise, I would make sure that the patient has adequate multimodal pain control, as pain can be a trigger for a carcinoid crisis.

Hypotension

Question 7

After the incision, the patient suddenly becomes hypotensive. What is your differential diagnosis? How would you manage this situation?

Answer 7

My differential includes hypovolemia secondary to blood loss, cardiogenic shock from acute arrhythmia, right ventricular failure, anaphylaxis, anesthetic overdose, and a carcinoid crisis.

I would quickly look at the VS to make sure the patient is not hypoxic, hypocarbic, or in a malignant arrhythmia. If the patient has been on preoperative octreotide treatment, hypotension is unlikely due to a carcinoid crisis. I would immediately open IV fluids wide open, give phenylephrine or vasopressin as a temporizing measure, and lighten the anesthetic.

I would communicate with the surgeons to see if there is more blood loss than expected, check the suction canister to determine estimated blood loss, and obtain an ABG to check hemoglobin, acid–base balance, and base excess—all of which could help me determine the cause of hypotension.

If I thought the hypotension was due to release of vasoactive mediators, I would give an additional 50–100 mcg octreotide every 5–10 minutes up to 1 mg and hydrocortisone. Aprotinin, a kallikrein inhibitor, has been used to treat hypotension refractory to octreotide as well.

Bronchospasm

Question 8

In the middle of case, you notice the patient's peak airway pressure suddenly rises. What do you do?

Answer 8

I would quickly check vital signs, making sure they were all stable. I would look at $EtCO_2$ to see if there are any acute changes.

I would then take the patient off the ventilator and begin manual ventilation to assess for airway compliance. I would also check my apparatus to ensure there is no kinking or occlusion of the circuit or ETT or ETT migration.

I would then increase the anesthetic depth in an effort to break the bronchospasm. If the peak airway pressure does not improve despite these measures and it is associated with skin flushing and manipulation of tumor by the surgeon, I would give an extra 100 mcg of octreotide bolus. I would administer albuterol as well if I was concerned for bronchospasms. I would be very cautious about bolusing epinephrine. Epinephrine can activate kallikrein in the tumor and lead to release of bradykinin, causing paradoxical vasodilation and worsening hypotension.

Question 9

What cardiac and metabolic disturbance would you expect to see from a patient on an octreotide infusion?

Answer 9

Octreotide may cause bradycardia, prolonged QT, and other conduction effects. Octreotide can cause glucose intolerance.

C. Postoperative Care

Pain

Question 1

How would you plan to manage the patient's pain postoperatively?

Answer 1

I would administer a fentanyl PCA for this patient, to help with pain control and to minimize histamine release. In addition, a neuraxial technique such as an epidural can be used, with caution, as hypotension can also precipitate a crisis.

Octreotide

Question 2

Your medical student asks if you want to discard the octreotide infusion, to simplify patient transfer to the ICU now that the patient is stable. What is your response?

Answer 2

There is no general agreement on the tapering of an octreotide infusion. The tapering regimen depends on severity of tumor, duration of surgery, type of procedure, the chances of undetected metastases, and residual effects of carcinoid tumor mediators. However, literature recommends tapering octreotide over a week postoperatively.

Placement

Question 3

The surgeon admits this patient to a regular-floor bed given the minimal blood loss and reported hemodynamic stability. What is your response?

Answer 3

I would kindly suggest that this patient be transferred to an ICU setting, as she would benefit from closer monitoring, for postoperative crisis is still possible. She will need at least 24 hours of invasive monitoring, and fluid management.

Suggested Readings

Bajwa SJ, Panda A, Kaur G. Carcinoid tumors: challenges and considerations during anesthetic management. *J Sci Soc.* 2015;42:132–137.

Castillo JG, Filsoufi F, Adams DH, Raikhelkar J, Zaku B, Fischer GW. Management of patients undergoing multivalvular surgery for carcinoid heart disease: the role of the anaesthetist. *Br J Anaesth.* 2008;101(5):618–626.

Mancuso K, Kaye AD, Boudreaux JP, et al. Carcinoid syndrome and perioperative anesthetic considerations. *J Clin Anesthesiol.* 2011;23:329–341.

Powell B, Al Mukhtar A, Mills GH. Carcinoid: the disease and its implications for anaesthesia. *Contin Educ Anaesth Crit Care Pain.* 2011;11(1):9–13.

Vaughan DJ, Brunner MD. Anesthesia for patients with carcinoid syndrome. *Int Anesthesiol Clin.* 1997;35(4):129–142.

9 Endocrine: Pheochromocytoma

Stanley Yuan and John Cooley

Stem 1

A 74-year-old, 56 kg, female presents for resection of an abdominal pheochromocytoma. She has had recurrent hypertensive episodes for the past month and has recently begun to experience palpitations and sweating.

Past medical history: Coronary artery disease

Past surgical history: Cardiac stents placed 5 years ago

Allergies: NKDA

Physical exam: Vital signs: pulse = 88 bpm, RR = 14, BP 121/76 mmHg, RA saturation 98%. Airway: Mallampati II, full cervical range of motion

Cardiovascular: Regular rate and rhythm

Pulmonary: Clear to auscultation

Hb = 14.2 g/dL, platelets = 240 K, K^+ = 3.3 mEq/L

A. Preoperative Evaluation

Medical Clearance

Question 1

How would you determine if this patient is optimized for surgery?

Answer 1

I would first perform a full history and physical. Initial assessment should include volume status, blood pressure trends, and symptoms of shortness of breath and chest discomfort. I would also want to know if she has been taking alpha blockers followed by beta-antagonist agents. This sequence is crucial to avoid hypertensive crisis from unopposed alpha action. According to the Roizen criteria, adequate blockade includes supine blood pressure under 160/90 mmHg, presence of orthostatic hypotension not greater than 80/45 mmHg, electrocardiogram without ST segment or T-wave changes, and no more than one premature ventricular contraction (PVC) every 5 minutes.

Question 2

How would you evaluate her cardiac status?

Answer 2

I would elicit from the patient what her baseline level of functioning is—specifically, whether she is able to walk up and down a flight of stairs without any discomfort, any recent episodes of chest pain, shortness of breath, or light-headedness. I would also look at a baseline EKG as well as the results of any echocardiogram or stress test that may have been recently done. If time permitted, I would want to talk to her cardiologist as well.

Question 3

Are there any additional workups you require the patient to have prior to surgery?

Answer 3

Currently, this patient has an elevated H/H, which is indicative of hypovolemia. I would also want serum electrolytes to assess renal function and glucose level, a chest X-ray to identify cardiomegaly or COPD, and a recent EKG to compare it to any old one. Since her coronary artery bypass graft (CABG) surgery was done 5 years ago, a recent echocardiogram and stress test are indicated.

Diagnosis

Question 4

How is pheochromocytoma diagnosed?

Answer 4

Pheochromocytomas are endocrine tumors that release catecholamines. With clinical suspicion, plasma metanephrine testing has the highest sensitivity for detecting pheochromocytomas. Elevated urinary vanillylmandelic acid (VMA) can also be used. With positive biochemical markers, computed tomography (CT) or magnetic resonance imaging (MRI) can be performed to localize the tumor with or without iodine 131–labeled metaiobenzyl-guanadine.

Question 5

What is the rule of 10s in pheochromocytomas?

Answer 5

The rule of 10s with pheochromocytomas is that 10% are bilateral, 10% are extrarenal, 10% are malignant, and 10% are familial.

Hypotension

Question 6

The patient suddenly becomes hypotensive and tachycardic preoperatively while changing into her gown. What do you do?

Answer 6

I would immediately check her vital signs and make sure the patient is adequately oxygenating and ventilating and that no malignant arrhythmia is developing with a 12 lead EKG. Assuming that was normal, I would rule out myocardial ischemia by asking targeted questions. If the patient is hypovolemic, I would administer 500 cc volume bolus with the patient placed supine on a stretcher. If no obvious underlying etiology was found, I would view it as a vasovagal response and treat it accordingly.

B. Intraoperative Management

Monitor

Question 1

How would you monitor this patient?

Answer 1

I would place the patient on standard ASA monitors with a five-lead electrocardiogram. A preinduction intra-arterial catheter is indicated to avoid blood pressure swings. With the nature of this surgery and fluid shift, central venous access is also important for both central venous pressure monitoring and the administrations of blood products and medications. I would also place a pulmonary arterial catheter or transesophageal echocardiography depending on her preoperative cardiac workup.

Induction

Question 2

How would you induce this patient?

Answer 2

Assuming a normal airway, I would preoxygenate this patient with 100% oxygen and perform a slow, controlled induction with fentanyl and etomidate and, once I saw I could mask ventilate, administer rocuronium. I would be looking at the arterial line reading during the induction and have pressors and dilators on standby to treat abrupt changes in blood pressure.

Question 3

During direct laryngoscopy, you are unable to visualize the vocal cords. What are you going to do?

Answer 3

I would mask ventilate with 100% oxygen and call for help. Assuming I am able to ventilate the patient, I would attempt direct laryngoscopy once again after repositioning the airway and switching blades. If I couldn't mask ventilate, I would place an LMA and attempt to ventilate the patient via the LMA.

Question 4

Are there other options besides general anesthesia for this surgery?

Answer 4

There are documented case reports of successful regional technique for open pheochromocytoma resection. One should focus on an anesthetic plan that is most comfortable and experienced. Communication with the surgical team is imperative. If this is an open anterior transabdominal approach, an epidural catheter can be inserted at around the T8 level for both intraoperative and postoperative analgesia.

Question 5

What medications, if any, would you avoid using during this case?

Answer 5

I would avoid drugs that would

1. Stimulate the tumor cells—succinylcholine by causing fasciculations, histamine-releasing drugs such as morphine and atracurium
2. Cause an increase in sympathetic activity—such as atropine, ketamine, and ephedrine

Hypertension

Question 6

Forty-five minutes into the case, during tumor manipulation the BP increases to 210/105 mmHg. How do you respond?

Answer 6

I would immediately look at the other vital signs and rule out hypoxia, hypercarbia, or a malignant rhythm while asking the surgeon to stop tumor manipulation. Highest on my differential is hypertension due to release of catecholamines from tumor manipulation. Thus, assuming the other vital signs are normal, I would immediately begin an infusion of sodium nitroprusside. Other agents that can be used are nitroglycerin and nicardipine, and if tachyarrhythmias are present, I would give esmolol.

Hypotension

Question 7

The patient is hypotensive immediately after the tumor is resected. What do you do?

Answer 7

Hypotension is common after tumor resection. I would first confirm the tracing on the intra-arterial line and ensure her other vital signs are stable. If the arterial line reading is true and other vital signs are stable, all vasodilators should be discontinued and the inhalational agent should be kept at minimal to ensure amnesia. I would order a stat H/H to assess intravascular volume and start volume resuscitation and aggressive inotropic support for cardiac and cerebral perfusion.

C. Postoperative Care

Delirium

Question 1

The patient develops altered mental status in the PACU. How do you differentiate delirium from postoperative cognitive dysfunction?

Answer 1

Delirium is characterized by the disturbance of perception, orientation, and psychomotor behavior and has a fluctuating clinical course. It usually develops within hours to days. Validation tests of delirium include the Confusion Assessment Method and the Delirium Rating Scale. Postoperative cognitive dysfunction (POCD) typically does not have a clear etiology. The patient presents with fluctuating mental status between postoperative days 1 and 3. The diagnosis of POCD requires baseline preoperative and postoperative neuropsychological testing, with independent risk of advanced age.

Question 2

The PACU nurse calls to inform you that the patient's serum glucose is 35 mg/dL. What do you do?

Answer 2

I would go and asses the patient at beside to make sure she is hemodynamically and neurologically stable. After confirming with another finger glucose check, I would start a 5% dextrose intravenous infusion with frequent finger sticks for the next 3 to 4 hours. Transient postoperative hypoglycemia episodes are not unusual in the PACU. This phenomenon is due to a surge of insulin sensitivity secondary to low serum catecholamine levels.

Hypotension

Question 3

In the PACU, do you anticipate hypertension or hypotension?

Answer 3

A small percentage of patients remain hypertensive in the postoperative period. If hypertension persists for more than a week, it may suggest an incomplete tumor resection. Most patients post-resection of pheochromocytoma experience episodes of hypotension instead. This is a result of persistent preoperative alpha-blockade. The best treatment at this point is probably crystalloid infusion, after ruling out potential cardiac issues.

Suggested Readings

Cole MG. Delirium in elderly patients. *Am J Geriatr Psychiatry.* 2004;12:7–21.

Fleisher LE, Beckman JA, Brown KA, et al. ACC/AHA 2009 guidelines on perioperative cardiovascular evaluation and care for noncardiac surgery: executive summary: a report of the American College of Cardiology/American Heart Association Task Force on Practice Guidelines. *Circulation.* 2009;116:1971–1996.

Lenders JW, Pacak K, Walther MM, et al. Biochemical diagnosis of pheochromocytoma: which test is best? *JAMA.* 2002; 287: 1427–1434.

10 Orthopedics: Shoulder Surgery

Sarah Madison

Stem 2

A 40-year-old male surfer is scheduled for arthroscopic rotator cuff repair at the ambulatory surgery center. He has a history of hypertension and chronic back pain. He has no past surgical history but claims his mother died during surgery from a "high fever." Vital signs are BP 166/89 mmHg, HR 65 bpm, RR 14, RA SpO_2 99%.

A. Preoperative Evaluation

Cardiac

Question 1

How would you evaluate this patient's cardiac status?

Answer 1

I would start with a focused history and physical. From the history, I would ask the patient about any history of heart attack, heart failure, or abnormal rhythms. Given his history of being a surfer, it is likely he lives an active lifestyle, but I would still inquire about his physical activity and any ischemic symptoms such as chest pain and shortness of breath. Then I would ask if he has had any diagnostic studies performed, such as an echocardiogram, exercise tolerance test, or screening EKG. On the physical exam, I would look for any signs of heart failure, such as JVD or pedal edema, as well as listen for regularity of rhythm and any murmurs. Finally, I would review any available tests such as EKG or echocardiogram and compare them to previous studies.

Question 2

How do you know his shoulder pain is not due to cardiac ischemia?

Answer 2

This would be determined on the basis of a thorough history and physical as well as a current EKG. If the shoulder pain is reproducible and consistent with an MRI lesion, then the pain is most likely stemming from the shoulder. However, if the patient has poor exercise tolerance with signs or symptoms of ischemia and a remarkable EKG, then the shoulder pain is likely cardiac in origin.

Hypertension

Question 3

How does this patient's history of hypertension affect your anesthetic management?

Answer 3

The patient's autoregulatory mechanism may be altered. My goal would be to keep his blood pressure within 20% of his baseline (or 30% if the patient is a candidate for an induced hypotensive technique).

Question 4

The surgeon is requesting "beach chair" positioning. How will this affect your hemodynamic goals?

Answer 4

I will have to take into account the placement of the noninvasive blood pressure cuff with respect to the patient's head. Cerebral perfusion may be lower than what the blood pressure cuff measures. Also, with venous pooling anticipated in the sitting position, I will have to ensure the patient is well hydrated and have pressors handy during positioning.

Question 5

Would you agree to a hypotensive technique to optimize visualization during arthroscopy?

Answer 5

Yes, as long as a recent stress test is normal, since I would need to drop the patient's blood pressure within 30% of his baseline.

Question 6

Other than for surgical exposure, what are some benefits of an induced hypotensive technique?

Answer 6

It decreases intraoperative blood loss up to 50% and shortens the surgical time by up to 1 hour.

Malignant Hyperthermia

Question 7

Should this case be done in an ambulatory surgery center or would you insist that it be done in the hospital?

Answer 7

This patient is a candidate for ambulatory surgery as long as a malignant hyperthermia (MH) cart is available and all the necessary precautions are taken for this case.

Question 8

Your resident asks you if you want to delay the case until a muscle biopsy is performed. How do you respond?

Answer 8

I would not delay the case for a muscle biopsy in this patient because it would not affect my anesthetic management. Based on the information given, I would treat this patient as MH susceptible and use a nontriggering technique.

Question 9

What precautions would you take in this patient given his family history?

Answer 9

First, I would flush out the anesthesia machine with 100% O_2 to remove any residual inhalational agents and remove any triggering agents from the OR, such as succinylcholine. I would make sure that I have infusion pumps ready for TIVA. I would have a fully stocked MH cart in the room and have a team meeting with the nurses and surgeon to discuss the MH protocol and what role each will play. I would have a central line and A-line setup handy and would contact the local hospital and ask them if they could reserve an ICU bed for us in the event that this patient develops MH during the case.

B. Intraoperative Management

Anesthesia

Question 1

Would you perform an axillary block for this patient?

Question 1

No. An axillary block would not cover the shoulder. I would perform an interscalene block preoperatively and offer the patient an ambulatory catheter. He may benefit from the opioid-sparing effects of a continuous interscalene catheter infusion.

Question 2

What is your choice of local anesthetic?

Answer 2

If the patient agreed to have a catheter placed, I would use 1.5% mepivacaine for quick onset; I can always re-dose the catheter. If he declined catheter placement, I would use a long-acting local anesthetic like ropivacaine 0.5% for prolonged analgesia. Adding epinephrine, clonidine, or dexamethasone might prolong the block even further.

Question 3

How would you counsel the patient on postoperative pain management?

Answer 3

I would encourage the patient to have an interscalene catheter placed because his chronic opioid use may make it difficult to control with oral opioids alone. A multimodal pain management regimen using a combination of oral opioids and local anesthetics, as well as adjuncts like acetaminophen or NSAIDs, are more effective than using opioids alone. If he opts for a single-injection block, I would counsel him to start taking his oral opioids before the block wears off.

Question 4

The patient says to you that his pinky finger doesn't feel numb at all and he thinks the block isn't working. What is your response?

Answer 4

This is a normal distribution of an interscalene nerve block. Ulnar sparing (the area of the pinky finger) is common with a properly placed interscalene block.

Question 5

The surgeon complains that the patient has complete sensation over the anterior deltoid. What is your response?

Answer 5

The anterior deltoid often receives innervation from the superficial cervical plexus, which is not always blocked with an interscalene block. I would test the interscalene block by testing terminal nerve distributions and deltoid strength. If the block was my sole anesthetic, I would perform a superficial cervical plexus block to supplement it.

Induction

Question 6

Let's assume you decided to supplement your regional block with a general anesthesia approach. How would you induce this patient?

Answer 6

Assuming the patient is NPO, has no other risk factors for aspiration, and has a truly favorable airway exam, I would perform a slow, controlled induction using lidocaine, fentanyl, propofol, and rocuronium. I would dose the propofol slowly and carefully to avoid hypotension.

Question 7

What monitors would you place on this patient?

Answer 7

I would place the standard ASA monitors. If the patient showed signs of autonomic instability with induction or positioning, I would have a low threshold for placing an arterial line.

Airway Management

Question 8

The surgeon asks if you can use a laryngeal mask airway (LMA) for this case. How do you respond?

Answer 8

An LMA can be used safely and offers the benefit of spontaneous ventilation in the seated position. However, I will not have access to the patient's airway during the case, and proper seating of an LMA may be challenging to maintain throughout the case. Thus, I would choose to have a secure airway using an endotracheal tube.

Question 9

Your colleague starts the case for you and places an LMA. Ten minutes into the surgery, the CO_2 machine alarms. You check the circuit and patient and find that the LMA has been dislodged. What is your next step?

Answer 9

After alerting the surgeon to the situation, turning on 100% oxygen, and ensuring the patient was adequately deep, I would call for help while attempting to reposition the LMA under the drapes while someone else prepared to mobilize the OR table back to the supine position. If my attempt was unsuccessful, I would place a mask on the patient with 100% O_2 until the table could be repositioned, assisting with ventilation as needed. After an adequate period of preoxygenation and a bolus of propofol, I would secure the patient's airway with an endotracheal tube.

Hypotension

Question 10

One hour into surgery, your machine alarms again. This time the heart rate is 23 bpm. The blood pressure cuff is cycling. What do you do?

Answer 10

I would immediately place the patient on 100% oxygen, check the EKG for a malignant arrhythmia, open the IV wide open, alert the surgeon and OR staff, and call for help and a crash cart while feeling for a pulse. If the pulse is weak, I would administer boluses of atropine and epinephrine to raise the

HR and BP while someone else starts repositioning the bed to prepare for chest compressions.

Question 11

What is the mechanism of the bradycardia?

Answer 11

There are multiple proposed mechanisms. In a patient undergoing general anesthesia, the most likely is activation of cardioinhibitory mechanoreceptors due to a reduction in preload with a hyperdynamic state (Bezold-Jarisch reflex). Other possibilities include carotid sinus hypersensitivity, orthostasis with venous pooling, and vasovagal response.

Question 12

Is there anything you could have done to prevent this complication?

Answer 12

It has been suggested that epinephrine added to the local anesthetic solution for brachial plexus block may predispose patients to initiate the Bezold-Jarisch reflex. Administration of a beta blocker may be protective; however, actual proof of this mechanism remains elusive.

C. Postoperative Management

The remainder of surgery is uneventful. The patient is extubated in the operating room and taken to the recovery room on oxygen facemask.

Pain

Question 1

The patient complains of pain in the PACU. How will you assess this?

Answer 1

I would go to the bedside and make sure the vital signs are stable. Next, I would ask the patient about the pain's location, severity, and possible radiation. Next, I would evaluate the block by testing pinprick sensation to determine if the block is providing adequate coverage to the surgical site.

Question 2

Is there anything you can do to optimize the block?

Answer 2

I can check the site to make sure the catheter is in place and no undue pressure is being placed on the extremity. Assuming it is intact, I would administer a bolus of local anesthetic through the interscalene catheter and monitor for any change in pain level.

Dyspnea

Question 3

Ten minutes after injecting local anesthetic through the interscalene catheter, the patient complains that he is short of breath. How will you assess him?

Answer 3

I would go to the bedside, assess the patient's vital signs, and make sure he is receiving oxygen by facemask. I would listen to breath sounds bilaterally, visualize chest excursion, and order a chest X-ray.

Question 4

Breath sounds are diminished on the left. Oxygen saturation is 96%. What is your differential diagnosis?

Answer 4

My differential would include pneumothorax and phrenic nerve palsy. Other less likely causes include unilateral atelectasis, pneumonia (PNA), and pulmonary embolism (PE).

Nausea

Question 5

The PACU nurse calls you to evaluate the patient for nausea. She mentions that the patient's face looks "droopy" and she is worried that he might have had a stroke. How will you assess the patient?

Answer 5

First, to evaluate the patient's nausea, I would look at the patient's vital signs, make sure he is receiving oxygen, and ask him about associated symptoms before prescribing an antiemetic. Then I would examine the patient to determine the etiology of the facial changes, looking specifically for ipsilateral ptosis (Horner's syndrome), which would be a side effect of the block and likely due to the bolus I just administered.

Question 6

What is your next step in management?

Answer 6

Horner's syndrome is an occasional side effect of interscalene block and does not pose a risk to the patient. Therefore, I would reassure the patient and the nurse that this is a normal finding and the symptoms will resolve in the next several hours.

Suggested Readings

Atchabahian A, Gupta R. *The Anesthesia Guide*. New York: McGraw-Hill;2013.

Dagli G, Güzeldemir EM, Acar VH. The effects and side effects of interscalene brachial plexus block by posterior approach. *Reg Anesth Pain Med*. 1998;23(1):87–91.

Song SY, Roh WS. Hypotensive bradycardic events during shoulder arthroscopic surgery under interscalene brachial plexus blocks. *Korean J Anesthesiol*. 2012;62(3):209–219.

11 Orthopedics: Hip Surgery in Aortic Stenosis

Ruchir Gupta

Stem 1

A 78-year-old female presents for emergent open reduction internal fixation (ORIF) of a hip fracture.

History of present illness: The patient fell off a chair in her nursing home. The fall was witnessed by a nurse's aide, who claimed she did not hit her head and was conscious the entire time.

Past medical history: Rheumatoid arthritis, hypertension (HTN), and aortic stenosis (AS).

EKG: No ST changes, LVH.

Physical exam: HR 111 bpm, BP 98/70 mmHg, RR 23, saturation 95% on 2 L.

The patient has severely limited neck movement.

Lungs are clear to auscultation.

Grade 4/6 systolic ejection murmur.

Labs: Hb 9 g/dL, Hct 27%, platelets 210 K.

A. Preoperative Evaluation

Hypertension

Question 1

Are you concerned about her history of HTN?

Answer 1

Yes, her history of HTN does concern me. Specifically, I am worried that her HTN may have shifted her autoregulation curve to the right, making it necessary for me to maintain her at a slightly higher mean arterial pressure (MAP) in order to maintain cerebral autoregulation, while risking further bleeding into the hip.

Question 2

What is the cerebral autoregulation curve? How does HTN affect it?

Answer 2

Perfusion to the brain is autoregulated by intrinsic mechanisms over a MAP of 50–150 mmHg. Below and above that range, the perfusion is no longer regulated and becomes dependent on actual blood flow. HTN shifts the curve, such that the range may be higher than the 50–150 mmHg range. Thus, maintaining a MAP of 50 mmHg may cause relative hypotension in a patient who has a history of HTN.

Cardiac Status

Question 3

How does the presence of aortic stenosis affect your anesthetic management?

Answer 3

My primary concern in patients with AS is the development of a myocardial infarction (MI) secondary to inadequate coronary perfusion pressure (CPP). Patients with AS need a high SVR to maintain the coronary perfusion according to the equation CPP = aortic diastolic pressure – left ventricular end diastolic pressure. Thus, if afterload (aDP) is compromised, CPP will decrease. My anesthetic management in this case would be to (1) maintain sinus rhythm because tachycardia not only increases myocardial oxygen demand but also decreases diastolic filling time in the coronary arteries, (2) maintain adequate preload, (3) maintain afterload because CPP is afterload dependent according to the equation, and (4) maintain contractility.

Question 4

What is the AS transvalvular gradient that would necessitate corrective valvular surgery?

Answer 4

50 mmHg

B. Intraoperative Management

Induction and Airway

Question 1

What invasive monitors would you use for this case?

Answer 1

I would place a preinduction A-line, central venous pressure CVP, and a TEE, with a cardiologist available for interpretation.

General vs. Regional

Question 2

Would you perform this case under general anesthesia or regional anesthesia? Why?

Answer 2

I would perform a general anesthetic technique for this case because of the emergent nature of the case, full-stomach status, anticipated hemodynamic instability, and history of a difficult airway.

Question 3

If you had to pick a regional technique for this case, would you decide on a spinal or an epidural?

Answer 3

A regional technique is not my first option. But if I had to pick one, I would perform an epidural in this patient as it allows for a greater degree of BP control. The sympathectomy caused by a dilute local anesthetic solution administered slowly through the epidural catheter will not be as great as the sympathectomy caused by a spinal.

Airway

Question 4

Assuming a general anesthetic technique is selected, how would you secure the airway?

Answer 4

After a careful airway examination, I would preoxygenate the patient with 100% oxygen, administer GI prophylaxis, and perform an awake fiber-optic intubation with an esmolol drip on standby.

Question 5

If you selected an awake fiber-optic technique, how would you anesthetize the airway?

Answer 5

I would topicalize the airway with nebulized lidocaine and block the superior laryngeal nerve by injecting local anesthetic at the greater cornu of the hyoid bone.

Question 6

As you introduce the fiber-optic scope into the pharynx, the BP rises to 220/130 mmHg. What do you do?

Answer 6

I would immediately withdraw the fiber-optic scope, assess the situation while ruling out hypoxia, and recheck the invasive and noninvasive blood pressure readings. If it appears that the patient is uncomfortable, I would administer more nebulized lidocaine. If the increased BP is due to anxiety, I would titrate in a very small amount of midazolam if reassuring the patient did not work. I would then reintroduce the fiber-optic scope and have an esmolol drip on standby.

Bone Cement Implantation Syndrome

Question 7

During the operation the patient suddenly becomes hypotensive. What will you do if the BP now reads 75/59 mmHg?

Answer 7

I would immediately look at the other vital signs and make sure the patient is not hypoxic, hypocarbic, or in a malignant arrhythmia. I would also recheck the A-line waveform, recycle the noninvasive BP cuff, check the H/H, and look at the TEE for heart chamber filling pressures. After placing the patient on 100% oxygen, I would then pressure bag the IV fluids and begin treatment with a pressor such as epinephrine/ephedrine if bradycardia is present and phenylephrine/norepinephrine if tachycardia is present. I would also communicate with the surgical team and examine the surgical field for active bleeding.

Question 8

The patient is not hypoxic. You look over at the surgical field and notice that the surgeon is cementing the prosthetic hip joint. How would this affect your further management?

Answer 8

Methyl methacrylate is a cement used in joint replacements that can cause hypotension usually 30–60 seconds after placement. Treatment involves mainly supportive measures with IV fluids and pressors.

Atrial Fibrillation

Question 9

The patient develops new-onset atrial fibrillation with a rapid ventricular response and a corresponding BP of 60/40 mmHg. What would be your immediate actions?

Answer 9

This is unstable atrial fibrillation. I would put the patient on 100% oxygen, feel for a carotid pulse, confirm the blood pressure readings, call for help, call for a code, and immediately perform synchronized cardioversion. I would also have amiodarone ready. I would send stat labs including ABG, H/H, electrolytes, cardiac enzymes, and a basic chemistry panel.

C. Postoperative Care

Extubation

Question 1

The surgery is now completed, which took 30 minutes less than anticipated. Are you going to extubate this patient?

Answer 1

No. This patient developed new-onset atrial fibrillation necessitating cardioversion and she suffered multiple bouts of hypotension. In addition, she has a difficult airway and has a diseased myocardium (AS). Thus, I would leave the patient intubated overnight and slowly wean the patient off once her other issues have stabilized. Had this been a routine case and the patient had been completely stable with no adverse events, I would consider extubation.

Question 2

Assuming you decided to leave the patient intubated, would you use propofol for sedation?

Answer 2

No, in this patient a propofol infusion could cause life-threatening hypotension given her history of AS. Thus, I would opt for an infusion of midazolam and fentanyl since they are more cardiac stable and provide better hemodynamics.

Postoperative Hypertension

Question 3

Two hours later you are paged to the PACU because the patient's BP has sharply risen to 210/110 mmHg. What are you going to do?

Answer 3

I would immediately go the patient's bedside and check vital signs to make sure the patient is not hypoxic, hypercarbic, or in a malignant arrhythmia. Assuming her other vital signs were normal, I would perform a focused history and physical to determine the etiology and treatment for her hypertension. From the history, I would check the anesthesia record and nurse's notes to see what medications had been given thus far. Because this patient has a history of hypertension, I would also check if she received her regularly scheduled dose of antihypertensive. From the physical, I would assess if the patient is sedated or is displaying signs of discomfort with the endotracheal tube. I would also see if the patient is sensitive to touch at the operative site. Finally, if everything was negative, I would administer a small bolus of esmolol/nitroglycerin depending on her heart rate.

Question 4

Would you order any labs?

Answer 4

It is unlikely that any lab work would help me narrow the differential. If I suspected hypoxia or acidosis as a possible cause and the pulse oximetry monitor and/or $EtCO_2$ monitor were not functioning properly, I would obtain an ABG.

Suggested Readings

Barash PG, Cullen BF, Stoelting RK, Cahalan M, Stock CM, eds. *Clinical Anesthesia*, 6th ed. Philadelphia, PA: Lippincott Williams & Wilkins; 2009.

Herrera A. Valvular heart disease. In: Hines R, Marschall K eds. *Stoelting's Anesthesia and Co-Existing Disease,* 5th ed. Philadelphia, PA: Churchill Livingstone; 2008.

Miller RD, Eriksson LI, Fleisher LA, Wiener-Kornish JP, Young WL, eds. *Miller's Anesthesia*. 7th ed. Philadelphia, PA: Churchill Livingstone Elsevier; 2010.

Morgan GE, Mikhail MS. *Clinical Anesthesiology*. New York: McGraw-Hill; 2006.

Yao F, Fontes ML, Malhotra V, eds. *Yao and Artusio's Anesthesiology: Problem-Oriented Patient Management*. 7th ed. Philadelphia, PA: Lippincott Williams & Wilkins; 2011.

12 Trauma: The Burn Patient

Ethan Kim and Ruchir Gupta

Stem 2

A 56-year-old 65 kg female was pulled out of her burning house. She is scheduled for an urgent open reduction and internal fixation of the right ankle. She has a history of HTN and hypercholesterolemia. Vital signs are pulse 105 bpm, BP 90/35 mmHg, RR 24 breaths, SpO_2 99% on 2 L supplemental oxygen, T 36.4°C. The patient is stridorous and combative and has a burn to the face, right upper extremity, and torso. She has a 20 g IV in the left arm.

A. Preoperative Evaluation

Initial Assessment

Question 1

What are your preoperative concerns regarding this patient?

Answer 1

I have several preoperative concerns about this patient. In terms of airway, I am concerned about her facial injuries, which may distort her anatomy and make for a difficult intubation. Additionally, based on the history given, it is likely she has experienced inhalation injury, which may lead to V/Q mismatch and also carbon monoxide poisoning. In terms of hemodynamics, burn patients are often severely hypovolemic. Since their capillaries are often leaky, one must be careful to resuscitate them with the appropriate fluid and rate as defined by the Parkland formula. In terms of her GI system, she is at risk for a Curling's ulcer, which may make her full stomach. Finally, I am concerned about her risk of infections because disruption of the skin barrier significantly increases her risk of full-blown sepsis.

Calculation for Percentage Burned

Question 2

The patient has burns to her right upper extremity, torso, and face. What percentage of her body is burned?

Answer 2

Thirty-six percent of her body is burned (9% for the upper extremity, 9% for face, and 18% for torso).

Question 3

If the patient had been a 1-year-old, what percentage burn would it be then?

Answer 3

Children have different proportions than adults. Thus, for a child the total percent would be 45% (9% for upper extremity, 18% for face, and 18% for torso).

Question 4

What if in addition to her current burns the patient also had a burn injury to her left upper extremity? How would that change the percentage burned?

Answer 4

Each upper extremity is 9% in the adult. Thus, in addition to her 36%, there would be an additional 9% area burned, for a total of 45%.

Carbon Monoxide Toxicity

Question 5

Are you satisfied with this patient's oxygen saturation?

Answer 5

No, I am not. Based on the information given, it seems very likely that she has suffered inhalation injury and is at risk for carbon monoxide poisoning. Such a condition would not be reflected on a standard pulse oximeter. To ascertain this, a co-oximeter can be used to truly measure the real oxyhemoglobin saturation.

Question 6

How does carbon monoxide affect the oxygen hemoglobin dissociation curve?

Answer 6

It shifts the curve downward and to the left.

Question 7

What other conditions shift the oxygen hemoglobin dissociation curve to the left? To the right?

Answer 7

The substances which shift the curve to the left are alkalosis, hypothermia, methemoglobin (met-Hb), fetal Hb, and decreased 2,3 DPG. Conversely, the substances shifting it to the right are acidosis, hyperthermia, and increased 2,3 DPG.

Question 8

The ABG of this patient shows pH 7.2, $PaCO_2$ 41, PaO_2 105, HCO_3^- 16. How would you interpret this ABG result and what can you do to improve this patient's condition?

Answer 8

This patient has uncompensated metabolic acidosis secondary to carbon monoxide poisoning. Carbon monoxide interferes with adequate oxygen delivery to tissues. I would administer 100% oxygen via facemask or ETT as it would decrease the half-life of carbon monoxide.

NPO Status

Question 9

The patient ate half a slice of pizza 10 hours ago. Will her burn injuries affect her NPO status?

Answer 9

Yes. This patient must be considered to have a full stomach because patients who experience major burns such as this patient are at risk for developing Curling's ulcers. Thus, this patient's gastric volume is greater than that of a normal individual who had been NPO for 10 hours.

Airway Evaluation

Question 10

How are you going to evaluate the patient's airway?

Answer 10

First, I would perform an external exam, looking for any distorting anatomical features. The presence of stridor in the patient reflects that airway soft tissue swelling has already taken place. Next, I would assess for any limitations in mouth opening and neck injuries and/or restriction of neck movement.

B. Intraoperative Management

Muscle Relaxation

Question 1

Can this patient receive succinylcholine for induction?

Answer 1

From the standpoint of the burn injuries, it is safe to administer succinycholine within the first 48 hours. After that time frame, succinylcholine can induce a massive lethal hyperkalemic response.

Airway

Question 2

How would you secure the airway?

Answer 2

I would prep and drape the neck for an emergency tracheotomy, have ENT on standby, and have the difficult-airway cart in the room with different sizes of ETT and LMAs. Then, I would perform a rapid sequence induction with etomidate and succinylcholine after administering GI prophylaxis.

Question 3

Can you perform awake fiber-optic intubation?

Answer 3

Yes, if the patient is hemodynamically stable and cooperative.

Monitoring

Question 4

Could you place an arterial line? Where? Pre- or postinduction?

Answer 4

I would place a preinduction A-line given that she is intravascularly depleted. Because there are burns to the arms, I would place a femoral arterial line and use the beat-to-beat monitoring of the BP to assist me during the case to avoid wide fluctuations in BP.

Fluid Therapy

Question 5

Your resident hangs a bottle of albumin during the case to improve the patient's volume status. Is this appropriate?

Answer 5

No, it is not. Colloids can worsen the hypovolemia by leaking through the capillaries into the extracellular space and increase the oncotic pressure of the extracellular space. This would further result in intravascular volume depletion.

Question 6

What would be your fluid resuscitation of choice? Why?

Answer 6

I would choose a crystalloid solution such as lactated Ringer's (LR) in this patient because it is not associated with metabolic acidosis, as is the case with normal saline (NS). Also, leakage of LR through the capillary membranes into the extracellular space will not affect the oncotic pressure the way it would with a colloid.

Question 7

What is the Parkland's formula?

Answer 7

Parkland's formula is a formula used to calculate the rate of fluid administration in a burn patient. It is 4 × % body surface area (BSA) burned × weight in kilograms. Half of this volume should be administered in the first 8 hours, ¼ in the second 8 hours, and the remaining ¼ in the last 8 hours.

C. Postoperative Care

Extubation Criteria

Question 1

Are you going to extubate this patient?

Answer 1

No. This patient is at high risk for airway swelling secondary to her baseline stridor, as well as other complications commonly associated with burns, such as sepsis, acute respiratory distress syndrome (ARDS), volume overload, and additional surgical procedures. In addition, burns to her torso may impair her ability to take adequate tidal volumes. Thus, I would keep this patient intubated and assess her airway swelling the following day by performing a "leak" test around the ETT. Assuming she has a leak and is able to breathe spontaneously, can take adequate tidal volumes without discomfort, and her other parameters are normal, I may extubate her in the ICU the following day.

ABG

Question 2

An ABG is repeated in the PACU and is as follows: pH 7.30, PCO_2 58 mmHg, PO_2 100 mmHg, HCO_3^- 20, O_2 saturation 99% on 100% FiO_2. Please interpret these findings.

Answer 2

This is metabolic acidosis with severe hypoxemia.

Question 3

Is the PO_2 adequate? Why or why not?

Answer 3

No, it isn't. A quick formula to determine an adequate PO_2 is 5 × FiO_2. Thus, in this patient, it should be 5 × 100 for a total of 500 mmHg. This patient has a PaO_2 of only 100 mmHg.

Oliguria

Question 4

What is the minimal urine output you would want for this patient? Why?

Answer 4

Minimum urine output for this patient should be kept to at least 0.5 mg/kg/hr. This is the minimum rate at which metabolic and nitrogenous wastes can be eliminated and normal ranges for electrolytes can be maintained.

Muscle Relaxation

Question 5

The patient returns 2 weeks later for an exploratory laparotomy. The surgeon informs you he will need extreme muscle relaxation for the case. What is your choice for muscle relaxation? Why?

Answer 5

I would choose a nondepolarizing muscle agent because a depolarizing agent such as succinycholine can lead to life-threatening hyperkalemia in the burn patient 24 hours after the burn. This risk is present whenever more than 10–20% of the BSA is burned (this patient has 36% burned). In terms of nondepolarizer I would administer rocuronium in larger than normal doses with re-bolusing as necessary. I will continue to monitor twitches because in any patient with greater than 25% BSA burn injuries, the dose of NDMR can be as high as 3–5 times normal.

Suggested Readings

Barash PG, Cullen BF, Stoelting RK, Cahalan M, Stock CM, eds. *Clinical Anesthesia*. 6th ed. Philadelphia, PA: Lippincott Williams & Wilkins; 2009.

Bittner EA, Shank E, Woodson L, Martyn J. Acute and perioperative care of the burn-injured patient. *Anesthesiology*. 2015;122(2):448–464.

Ryan CM, Schoenfeld DA, Thorpe WP, et al. Objective analysis of the probability of death from burn injuries. *N Engl J Med*. 1998;338 (6):362–366.

13 Trauma: Multisystem Injury

Dion M. McCall, Molly Amin,
and Michal Gajewski

Stem 1

A 41-year-old, 50 kg female presents to the trauma suite for an ORIF of a closed right humerus fracture. The patient was a restrained driver in a motor vehicle accident (MVA).

Past medical history: Hypertension

Physical exam: Vital signs: HR 110 bpm, BP 90/60 mmHg, RR 24, O_2 saturation 96% on nonrebreather mask

Airway: Mallampati II

Cardiovascular: Tachycardic, bruises on left chest

Respiratory: Decreased breath sounds on left side

Abdomen: diffuse tenderness with ecchymosis on the left flank

Imaging studies: Head CT—negative for any injuries

Hb = 10.1 g/dL, platelets = 240 K, WBC = 14 K cells per mcL

A. Preoperative Management

Question 1

What is the Glasgow Coma Scale?

Answer 1

The Glasgow Coma Scale (GCS) is the most common scoring system used to describe the level of consciousness in a person after suffering a traumatic brain injury. In the GCS, three indices (eye opening, verbal response, and motor response) are used to produce a combined value between 3 and 15 for any given individual. A score below 9 indicates severe brain injury; between 9 and 12, moderate injury; and 13 or greater, minor injury.

Question 2

What is the role of an abdominal paracentesis in a trauma patient? What is a FAST examination (focused assessment by sonography for trauma)?

Answer 2

Abdominal paracentesis is performed when intra-abdominal bleeding is suspected in a hemodynamically unstable patient with a high-risk mechanism of injury. The paracentesis is a means of rapidly diagnosing intra-abdominal injury requiring an exploratory laparotomy.

Focused **A**ssessment by **S**onography in **T**rauma (FAST):

This is a technique to quickly diagnose hemorrhage in a trauma patient using ultrasound. It generally takes less than 3 minutes and looks at four different views: right upper quadrant (RUQ), left upper quadrant (LUQ), subxiphoid, and suprapubic. The goal is to identify blood accumulation in these areas.

Question 3

How would you assess this patient's fluid status?

Answer 3

I would assess the fluid status by performing a focused history and physical examination. From the history, I would review the paramedic's notes as well as the ER notes to see if her vitals have been stable or are gradually getting worse. I would also look to see what fluids or blood products she has received since her injury. From the physical exam I would look for any foci of bleeding and assess her clothes for any blood on them. I would also check any suction canisters to see if they have any blood. I would look at her mucus membranes, skin turgor, and 2-second capillary refill to assess her current volume status. Finally, I would order a stat basic metabolic panel (BMP) and ABG to assess for signs of hypovolemia, which may manifest as hypernatremia and/or acidosis secondary to lack of tissue perfusion.

Question 4

Would you order any additional labs for this patient?

Answer 4

Yes, in addition to the CBC, I would also want electrolytes, coagulation profile, ABG, and a type and cross.

Question 5

What is the definition of shock?

Answer 5

Shock is an abnormality of the circulatory system that results in inadequate organ perfusion and tissue oxygenation, ultimately leading to anaerobic metabolism.

Question 6

What are the different types of shock? Describe each one.

Answer 6

Hypovolemic shock occurs secondary to a decrease in intravascular volume leading to decreased venous return and subsequent reduced stroke volume and cardiac output. Hypovolemic shock can be secondary to hemorrhage or increased losses of body fluid.

Cardiogenic shock results from decreased cardiac output due to intrinsic myocardial dysfunction. Myocardial infarction, decompensated CHF, arrhythmia, and cardiomyopathy are examples of conditions causing cardiogenic shock.

Obstructive shock occurs when mechanical factors impede inflow or outflow to the heart, as in pericardial tamponade, tension pneumothorax, or pneumomediastinum.

Distributive shock manifests when decreased or absent vasomotor function is significant enough to decrease venous return and stroke volume. Neurogenic and septic shock are included in this class. In *neurogenic shock* a CNS injury, nitrates, opioids, or sympatholytic drugs lead to a loss of vasomotor tone, whereas in *septic shock* bacterial toxins stimulate the release of vasoactive mediators.

B. Intraoperative Management

Question 1

What type of monitoring are you going to use on this patient?

Answer 1

I would place standard ASA monitors along with an arterial line, a central line, and a Foley catheter.

Question 2

What kind of IV access would you require?

Answer 2

For IV access, I would use a central line and also place multiple large-bore PIVs.

Question 3

How does shock affect anesthetic management of this patient?

Answer 3

Hemorrhagic shock potentiates the effects of the anesthetic on the brain, leading to at least a 25% decrease in MAC. As the patient is already intubated, I would use one of the least soluble inhalation agents, such as Desflurane, for maintenance of anesthesia at concentrations less than 1 MAC to allow for rapid titration if severe hemodynamic instability occurs.

Question 4

Are you concerned about the patient having postoperative recall when running less than 1 MAC for maintenance of anesthesia?

Answer 4

Yes, I am; however, my primary goal is to maintain adequate organ perfusion, at least until there is surgical hemorrhage control. In order to minimize the chances of recall I would supplement with opioids and benzodiazepines as tolerated and use scopolamine if available.

Question 5

How would you address the cervical neck concerns of a trauma patient?

Answer 5

These patients tend to come straight to the OR with a cervical collar in place. It would be prudent for me to speak with the patient as he or she can verbalize neck pain and even demonstrate neck movements. This would help me determine whether to employ an awake fiber-optic technique instead of an RSI. If I had negative neck films on anteroposterior (AP) view, lateral view, and odontoid view, my concerns would be diminished.

Question 6

How would you induce anesthesia?

Answer 6

Assuming the patient has a normal airway and recognizing that she has a full stomach, I would preoxygenate with 100% O_2, remove the neck collar while having an assistant maintain in-line stabilization, and proceed with a rapid sequence induction. I would induce with etomidate and succinylcholine while applying cricoid pressure. I would also make sure I have the difficult-airway cart in the room with various sized ETT and LMAs lubed and ready for any emergency situation.

Question 7

Five minutes after induction the patient's blood pressure drops to 60/30 mmHg while peak airway pressure increases to 25 cm H_2O. What is your differential diagnosis?

Answer 7

My primary concern would be a tension pneumothorax because of her initial decreased breath sounds on the left. Since the patient has suffered an MVA and has ecchymosis over the left flank, I would also consider a hemothorax. Other possibilities could be anaphylactic reaction to a recently administered drug, a mainstem intubation, bronchospasm, kinked ETT, ETT obstruction due to a mucus plug, and pulmonary edema.

Question 8

The patient continues to bleed excessively. A recent ABG shows a Hgb of 5.7 g/dL. What is a massive blood transfusion? Would you initiate it at this time? Why or why not?

Answer 8

Yes, I would. A *massive blood transfusion* is defined as replacement of greater than one blood volume in 24 hours or greater than 50% of blood volume in 4 hours. Considering the patient's Hgb is 5.7 g/dL and the bleeding is ongoing, the massive transfusion will help maintain tissue perfusion and oxygenation by restoring blood volume, while blood component therapy will help correct any coagulopathic conditions.

Question 9

What is the ratio of packed red blood cells to fresh frozen plasma to platelets (PRBCs:FFP:Plt) you want to use during a massive blood transfusion?

Answer 9

Patients with severe trauma who undergo massive blood replacement and develop secondary coagulopathy have improved survival when the ratio of transfused PRBCs to fresh frozen plasma to platelets is closer to 1:1:1. Thus, I would start the transfusion on the basis of this guideline and then use my clinical judgment to further guide therapy.

Question 10

What are some of the complications associated with a massive blood transfusion?

Answer 10

Complications of massive blood transfusion include thrombocytopenia, coagulation factor depletion, hypocalcemia, hyperkalemia, acid–base disturbances, transfusion-related lung injury (TRALI), and acute respiratory distress syndrome (ARDS).

C. Postoperative Management

Question 1

Would you extubate this patient? If so, how?

Answer 1

Given the patient's history of blunt chest trauma, risk of pulmonary contusion, and fluid shifts from an extensive resuscitation effort, I would leave the patient intubated. I would re-evaluate the patient for extubation when she is more hemodynamically stable and the pulmonary contusion has had time to declare itself.

Question 2

What are your extubation criteria?

Answer 2

I would evaluate the patient for an adequate respiratory drive, respiratory muscle strength, and a cough reflex to clear secretions.

I would also look at gas exchange, making sure that there is an adequate PaO_2/FiO_2 ratio >150–200. I would also look for an appropriate pH (pH ≥7.25) and $PaCO_2$ during spontaneous ventilation.

Other items that are necessary include a RR <35, vital capacity >15 mL/kg, NIF > −20 cmH_2O, tidal volume >5 mL/kg, and a minute ventilation <10 L/min.

Question 3

You decide to keep the patient intubated and transfer her to the ICU. The patient's temp is 33.5°C. What are some effects of hypothermia?

Answer 3

While mild hypothermia decreases the metabolism of most drugs, wound infection is the most common serious complication, owing to impaired immune function and decreased blood flow cutaneously. Hypothermia also reduces platelet function and decreases the activation of the coagulation cascade, while moderate to severe hypothermia can lead to cardiac arrhythmias and death.

Shivering from hypothermia causes significant increases in oxygen consumption, CO_2 production, and cardiac output.

Question 4

How would you treat the hypothermia?

Answer 4

Hypothermia should be treated with a forced-air warming device and/or with warming lights or heating blankets that will help raise the patient's body temperature to normal. Use of heating fluids to near 37°C also helps to prevent hypothermia.

Question 5

You are paged to the ICU because over the course of several hours, the patient's hemodynamics have deteriorated. CVP is now 22 mmHg, PA 46/25 mmHg, CI 1.5 L/min/m^2 with minimal urine output. What do you suspect is happening? How would you evaluate?

Answer 5

I would suspect an acute cardiac tamponade and would look for Becks triad of hypotension, jugular-venous distension, and muffled heart sounds. An echocardiogram would be very useful to look for pericardial fluid and an EKG may show ST-segment changes and low-voltage QRS complexes. Sometimes a pericardial rub can also be heard with a stethoscope.

Question 6

How would you treat this?

Answer 6

I would immediately inform the surgeon, open the IV fluids wide open, support the vital signs with dopamine, and prepare this patient for transfer to the OR for an emergent pericardial window. If the surgeon believes that the patient is a candidate for a bedside pericardiocentesis, I would arrange for IV anesthetic agents as well as resuscitative medicines to be placed next to the patient's bed.

Question 7

Seventy-two hours postoperatively, you notice that the patient has developed progressive hypoxemia. A chest X-ray shows bilateral "whiteout" of both lung fields. PaO_2 is 64 mmHg on FiO_2 of 70%. What is your diagnosis?

Answer 7

This patient is most likely in ARDS, a form of acute respiratory failure in which the alveolar capillary membrane becomes damaged and more permeable to intravascular fluid. Its diagnosis is usually dependent on signs of acute, refractory hypoxemia, diffuse infiltrates consistent with pulmonary edema, and a pulmonary capillary wedge pressure less than 18 mmHg. These patients usually have a PaO_2/FIO_2 ratio of less than 200 mmHg.

Question 8

Will you administer positive end-expiratory pressure (PEEP)? How would using PEEP help?

Answer 8

Yes. PEEP can help improve oxygenation by preventing alveolar collapse at end expiration and therefore increase lung volume. This would help improve V/Q matching.

Suggested Readings

Barash PG, Cullen BF, Stoelting RK, Cahalan M, Stock CM, eds. *Clinical Anesthesia*. 6th ed. Philadelphia, PA: Lippincott Williams & Wilkins; 2009.

Morgan GE, Mikhail MS, eds. *Clinical Anesthesiology*. New York: McGraw-Hill; 2006.

Smith TC, Marini JJ. Impact of PEEP on lung mechanics and work of breathing in severe airflow obstruction. *J Appl Physiol*. 1988;65(4):1488–1499.

14 Trauma: Traumatic Brain Injury

Ruchir Gupta

Stem 2

A 53-year-old, 5'6", 120 kg male presents to the OR for emergent craniotomy. He is somnolent, spontaneously breathing, and speaking incoherently. On physical examination, he has a swollen right arm, ecchymosis into the periorbital area, multiple facial fractures, and several loose teeth. A relative informs staff that the patient has chronic hypertension and bipolar disorder. NS is running through an 18 g IV on the left antecubital arm. Vital signs are HR 129 bpm, BP 180/110 mmHg, RR 28, SpO_2 94% on a nonrebreathable mask. Hb = 9.1 mg/dL.

A. Preoperative Evaluation

Trauma

Question 1

The patient has been NPO for at least 8 hours. Is this information helpful?

Answer 1

No. Acute trauma victims are assumed to have a full stomach because the stress response from the trauma decreases the parasympathetic nervous system activity and therefore GI motility is diminished. Additionally, it is unclear if this patient has any comorbid conditions that may predispose him to aspiration, such as hiatal hernia, diabetic induced gastroparesis, or GERD.

Glasgow Coma Scale

Question 2

As you begin to examine the patient you notice that he opens his eye only to pain, is uttering incomprehensible sounds, and is displaying a decorticate response. What is his Glasgow Coma Scale (GCS) score?

Answer 2

His GCS score is 7. His eye opening to pain is a score of 2, the uttering of incomprehensible sounds is also a 2, and the decorticate response has a score of 4, for a total of 7.

Question 3

What is meant by a decorticate response?

Answer 3

A *decorticate response* is defined as abnormal flexion to painful stimuli.

Intracranial Hypertension

Question 4

What is the difference between an epidural hematoma and a subdural hematoma?

Answer 4

There are several differences between an epidural and a subdural hematoma. First, epidural hematomas usually occur from a tear in the mid-meningeal artery and collect between the skull and the dura. Subdural hematomas occur after a traumatic brain injury, as seen in this patient, and occur between the dura and subarachnoid layers. In epidural hematomas, there is a lucid interval followed by a loss of consciousness, whereas in subdural hematoma there is no such interval. On a CT epidurals appears as a biconvex shape, whereas a subdural appears as a concave shape.

Substance Abuse

Question 5

A toxicology screen done in the ER reveals evidence of cocaine abuse. How does this affect your anesthetic management?

Answer 5

Cocaine inhibits the reuptake of several substances that are involved in the regulation of sympathetic nervous system. Chronic abusers will often display labile BP, severe HTN, and possibly difficult vascular access. Acute intoxication can result in ventricular fibrillation, seizures, and catastrophic MI. Thus, I would:

1. Have a preinduction arterial line to closely monitor the BP and a 5 lead EKG to monitor for myocardial ischemia.
2. Have infusions of nitroprusside and esmolol ready in case I need to rapidly lower the BP.
3. Make sure I have at least two large-bore IVs and if not used, place a central line.
4. Use only direct-acting agents such as phenylephrine and avoid indirect-acting agents such as ephedrine because these patients may display an exaggerated response to indirect-acting agents.
5. Use universal precautions for myself and other health care workers because he may have HIV or hepatitis C from IV drug use.

Question 6

What if the patient was a chronic alcoholic? How would that affect your anesthetic care?

Answer 6

From a cardiac standpoint, chronic alcoholism can lead to cardiomyopathy. Thus, I would avoid agents that are direct myocardial depressants. From a GI standpoint, cirrhosis or fatty liver may be present, depending on the severity of the alcoholism. Thus, I would try to avoid using drugs that undergo hepatic clearance. I would also avoid any neuraxial techniques because the PT might be elevated. These patient may have gastritis, so I would use an RSI to secure the airway. From a neurological standpoint, higher MAC values may be needed to keep the patient anesthetized. Thus I would administer higher than normal MAC values to the patient.

Cervical Spine

Question 7

Can a plane X-ray be used to clear the cervical spine?

Answer 7

No. An X-ray alone is not sufficient to clear a trauma victim's cervical spine because soft tissue injuries, such as ligament damage, cannot be seen on a plane X-ray.

Question 8

So how would you clear this patient's cervical spine?

Answer 8

There are four major components to cervical spine clearance:

1. Age over 4 years
2. Absence of cervical tenderness
3. Absence of neurological deterioration and paresthesias
4. Lack of distracting injuries

If these conditions were not met, I could use cervical radiographs with AP views with open-mouth odontoid and lateral views including T1. However, even if these were normal, I would still need a cervical MRI to determine if there is any ligamentous injury that wasn't apparent on the X-rays.

B. Intraoperative Management

Induction

Question 1

How would you induce this patient?

Answer 1

This patient presents as a full stomach and as a potentially difficult airway secondary to his multiple facial fractures that may distort anatomy. In addition, I would want to avoid gagging and bucking because that can worsen the ICP in this patient with a head injury. Thus, after prepping and draping the neck for an emergent tracheostomy and having the tracheostomy kit open, with ENT on standby, I would perform an RSI with in-line neck stabilization using etomidate and succinycholine.

Question 2

What monitors would you place on this patient?

Answer 2

I would place the standard ASA monitors; central line for fluid management and possible venous air embolism treatment; and an A-line for continuous BP monitoring, serial ABGs, and H/H assessment.

Question 3

Your resident asks you to use ketamine to maintain spontaneous ventilation in the patient during induction. How do you respond?

Answer 3

I would inform the resident that ketamine is contraindicated in a patient with increased ICP and can worsen the BP if cocaine is already in his system.

Question 4

Can you use N_2O for maintenance in this patient?

Answer 4

I would avoid using N_2O in this patient because I want to avoid any risk of expanding unknown air pockets within the cranium that would worsen the ICP. In addition, I want to maintain this patient on 100% FiO_2 given the nature of his injuries. Administration of N_2O would inevitably cause me to lower the FiO_2.

Question 5

You determine that this patient has an elevated ICP. What steps can you take to lower the ICP in this patient prior to surgical incision?

Answer 5

There are several steps that can be taken. First, I could hyperventilate the patient to a $PaCO_2$ of 30 mmHg and elevate the head of the bed 15–30 degrees to promote venous drainage. Next, I would administer mannitol and furosemide as tolerated by the BP, assuming the blood–brain barrier (BBB) was intact. I could also loosen the neck collar to further promote venous drainage and prevent any venous engorgement of the cranium. Finally, I could consider using a barbiturate to reduce the ICP and decrease the cerebral metabolic rate of oxygen ($CMRO_2$).

Blood Products

Question 6

One hour into the case, the BP suddenly drops to 70/30 mmHg. What will you do?

Answer 6

I will immediately look at the vital signs and ensure the patient is not hypoxic, hypercarbic, or in a malignant arrhythmia. I would also recheck the position of my A-line transducer and cycle the NIBP to ensure this is an accurate reading. I would also communicate with the surgeon and look at the surgical field to assess for severe hemorrhaging. Assuming all of the other vital signs are normal, I would open the fluids wide and administer small boluses of a vasopressor such as phenylephrine as a temporizing measure until a definitive diagnosis can be made.

Question 7

You look at the patient's other vital signs and notice that the $EtCO_2$ tracing is at zero. What do you think is going on?

Answer 7

The highest possibility on my list would be a venous air embolism, because hypotension with a loss of $EtCO_2$ in the presence of exposed sinuses places this patient at risk. Other possibilities include a PE, fat embolism, disconnected ETT, MI, and a malignant arrhythmia (such as ventricular fibrillation [Vfib]).

C. Postoperative Care

Polyuria

Question 1

You are paged stat to the PACU because the patient's Na is 124 mEq/L. What is your differential diagnosis?

Answer 1

Considering the nature of this patient's injury, my differential would be syndrome of inappropriate antidiuretic hormone (SIADH), overhydration, and cerebral salt wasting syndrome (CSWS).

Question 2

What lab tests would you tell your resident to obtain, to distinguish CSWS from SIADH?

Answer 2

I would tell the resident to obtain a urine osmolarity test as well as the hourly urine output for the previous 24 hours. In a patient with SIADH, the urine osmolarity is high, whereas in the CSWS patient it would be low or normal. In addition, CSWS patients exhibit polyuria, whereas patients with SIADH will have decreased urine output.

ARDS

Question 3

On postoperative day (POD) #1, the patient develops bilateral infiltrates on chest X-ray and has a PaO_2 of 75 mmHg on 100% FiO_2. What are the criteria for diagnosing ARDS?

Answer 3

The criteria for diagnosing ARDS are as follows:

- Identifiable etiology
- Acute onset
- Pulmonary artery wedge pressure ≤18 mmHg or absence of clinical evidence of left atrial hypertension
- Bilateral infiltrates on chest X-ray
- PaO_2/FiO_2 ratio ≤200

Question 4

What would you call it if the PaO_2/FiO_2 ratio were ≤300 but >200 mmHg?

Answer 4

In that case, it would be called acute lung injury.

Question 5

How would you treat the patient in this situation?

Answer 5

Assuming this is ARDS, treatment is usually supportive with mechanical ventilation, treatment of the etiology with antibiotics if indicated, PEEP to recruit collapsed alveoli, diuretics, and an FiO_2 of 50% or less to prevent oxygen toxicity.

Suggested Readings

Barash PG, Cullen BF, Stoelting RK, Cahalan M, Stock CM, eds. *Clinical Anesthesia*. 6th ed. Philadelphia, PA: Lippincott Williams & Wilkins; 2009.

Miller RD, Eriksson LI, Fleisher LA, Wiener-Kornish JP, Young WL, eds. *Miller's Anesthesia*. 7th ed. Philadelphia, PA: Churchill Livingstone Elsevier; 2010.

Yao F, Fontes ML, Malhotra V, eds. *Yao and Artusio's Anesthesiology: Problem-Oriented Patient Management*. 7th ed. Philadelphia, PA: Lippincott Williams & Wilkins; 2011.

15 Urology: TURP Syndrome

Mark Slomovits

Stem 2

A 76-year-old male presents for transurethral resection of the prostate (TURP).

Past medical history: DM, HTN, and hypercholesterolemia.

Medications: Metformin, HCTZ, and simvastatin.

All: Percutaneous nephrostomy (PCN).

Physical exam: Vital signs: BP 112/86 mmHg, RR 16, HR 67 bpm, SPO_2 97% on RA. On physical exam he has a Mallampati II airway with full cervical range of motion. The remainder of the physical exam is unremarkable.

Labs: K 3.4 mEq/L, creatinine 1.3 mg/dL.

A. Preoperative Evaluation

Assessment of Comorbidities

Question 1

What preoperative information would you want to know before taking this patient to the OR?

Answer 1

Based on the information given, I would want to know more specific details about this patient's chronic conditions. With respect to his diabetes, I would want to know if it is well controlled, what this patient's HbA1C level is, and whether he has any signs or symptoms of any complications from uncontrolled diabetes, such as neuropathy, vasculopathy, or nephropathy. In terms of his history of hypertension, I would want to know if it has been well controlled and whether he has any complications from long-standing hypertension, such as nephropathy or left ventricular hypertrophy. With regard to labs, I would want a CBC to rule out anemia of chronic disease and assess platelet levels, a metabolic panel to determine blood glucose with a BUN/creatinine to assess renal function, and a baseline EKG.

Question 2

You obtain an EKG that reveals left ventricular hypertrophy (LVH) and Q waves in the lateral leads. How would you proceed?

Answer 2

The ventricular hypertrophy may be an indication of several conditions, but specific to this patient it may indicate long-standing hypertension. The Q waves are indicative of past cardiac ischemia or an old myocardial infarction and would lead me to assume that the patient has some indolent coronary disease. Furthermore, the presence of coronary disease is worsened in the setting of LVH because of a greater baseline myocardial demand. If available, I would want to compare this EKG to an old one to see if these changes are new. If so, I would insist on the patient undergoing further noninvasive cardiac testing, such as a stress test or an echocardiogram, before the procedure can be performed safely.

Question 3

Assuming the EKG findings are stable chronic changes, how would you proceed if the platelet count is noted to be 99,000 and the hemoglobin is 9.8 g/dL?

Answer 3

I would want to trend the patient's labs with older ones to determine if it is an acute or chronic condition. Given this patient's history of diabetes, this could very well be anemia of chronic disease. Assuming it was chronic, I would type and cross this patient and have blood available before the start of the procedure. If this was acute, I would attempt to determine what the possible cause could be. If the patient's low platelet count was chronic and the patient was otherwise asymptomatic, I would not be concerned. If this was an acute drop, I would want to investigate further and determine the cause.

Laser

Question 4

The surgeon suggests that he can resect the prostate with reduced bleeding using laser therapy rather than electrocautery. What concerns, if any, would you have with using the laser intraoperatively?

Answer 4

Laser use in clinical settings is dependent on laser wavelength, energy density, and tissue absorption. Variations in these factors affect the depth and destructiveness of the signal; a proper laser would need to be chosen that penetrates the prostatic tissue to the appropriate depth but also has poor tissue absorption because of the potential for damage to surrounding tissue that is also exposed to the irrigation fluid. There is a risk of fire in the OR if the laser is mishandled. This can be avoided if the laser is kept in standby mode when not in use. Finally, all personnel (and the patient) should wear proper goggles that are specifically rated to filter out the wavelength of the laser, to avoid eye damage.

B. Intraoperative Management

Monitoring

Question 1

What monitors would you want to use for this patient's procedure? Why?

Answer 1

In addition to the standard ASA monitors, I would also have an arterial line in place. An arterial line is essential as the patient has multiple cardiac risk factors. Also, this particular surgery is associated with the risk for massive intravascular volume absorption and subsequent hemodynamic instability.

Regional vs. General Anesthesia

Question 2

Would you perform a general anesthetic or regional technique in this patient?

Answer 2

Assuming this patient has no contraindications to a regional, such as a coagulopathy or patient refusal, I would choose to perform this case under a spinal anesthetic because I would want an awake patient, which allows me to assess the mental status during the case.

Question 3

What are the advantages and disadvantages of each?

Answer 3

The benefits of a neuraxial technique in this patient are the following:

1. Ability to monitor mental status in anticipation of possible development of the TURP syndrome, bladder perforation, or myocardial infarction
2. Reduced need for systemic opioids for postoperative pain control
3. Avoidance of instrumenting the airway with the associated hemodynamic fluctuations of an induction

The disadvantages of a regional technique are the following:

1. Possibility of intraoperative anxiety and awareness in the awake patient

2. Development of a high spinal/epidural necessitating emergent control of airway and maintenance of hemodynamics
3. Inadequate level of blockade (below desired T10)

With respect to general anesthesia, the benefits are as follows:

1. Secure airway
2. Lack of awareness and intraoperative anxiety
3. Can ensure proper depth of anesthesia without worry about level of block

The disadvantages are as follows:

1. Inability to monitor mental status
2. Increased need for systemic opioids for postoperative pain
3. Necessity of induction with associated hemodynamic fluctuations

Question 4

If you choose a neuraxial approach, which type of regional block would you offer? What level of anesthetic blockade would you wish to achieve?

Answer 4

I would choose a single-shot spinal and attempt a T10 level.

TURP

Question 5

You perform an uncomplicated bupivacaine spinal anesthetic, achieving a T10 level. Thirty minutes into the procedure the patient complains of nausea and progressively becomes restless and disoriented. What is your differential? What would you do?

Answer 5

I would be concerned about cardiac ischemia, cerebral vascular event, hypoxia, pulmonary edema, hyperglycemia, or bladder perforation. However, my immediate concern is the onset of TURP syndrome. I would immediately look at the vital signs and rule out hypoxia, hypercarbia, hypotension, or a malignant arrhythmia. I would also notify the surgeon of the events and request that they terminate irrigating immediately. I would then control the airway by inducing and intubating the patient and placing him on continuous mechanical ventilation. Finally, I would send off an ABG test to evaluate for the serum sodium and glucose values.

Question 6

What would be the properties of an ideal irrigating fluid for a TURP procedure?

Answer 6

The ideal irrigating solution should be:

1. Isotonic—to prevent hemolysis encountered in hypotonic solutions
2. Electrically inert—to prevent interference with electrocautery and dissemination of electrical current
3. Transparent—to allow proper visualization by the surgeon
4. Nontoxic—due to risk of significant systemic absorption

Question 7

What is TURP syndrome?

Answer 7

TURP syndrome describes a complex of symptoms resulting from acute volume expansion and dilutional hyponatremia manifesting as hypertension (followed by hypotension), refractory bradycardia, and neurological symptoms that range from vague to severe and may ultimately result in lethargy, tonic clonic seizures, coma, and death.

Additional info:

The prostatic urethra is rich in venous sinuses that become exposed during the course of prostatic resection. Since the resection is performed using a cystoscope, the surgical field must be kept clear of resected debris, which is accomplished using continuous fluid irrigation. The exposure of the prostatic sinuses to irrigation fluid (particularly hypotonic fluids) results in systemic absorption, which leads to a dilutional hyponatremia. The absorption volume of irrigating fluid is dependent on the number of open sinuses, the flow rate of the fluid, the hydrostatic pressure of the fluid, the venous pressure at the sinus–irrigant interface, and the duration of the resection. The onset of hyponatremia depends on the rate of the fluid absorption and also on the osmolality of the fluid, where lower-osmolality irrigating fluid will contribute to a more rapid development of hyponatremia.

Bladder Perforation

Question 8

Could this be due to a bladder perforation?

Answer 8

Bladder perforation is certainly a possibility because one would still see nausea and vomiting and generalized restlessness, as demonstrated with this patient. However, classically, there is also shoulder pain from diaphragmatic irritation because most bladder perforations are extraperitoneal.

Hyponatremia

Question 9

You successfully intubate the patient and initiate mechanical ventilation. An ABG sample shows pH 7.46, pCO_2 22 mmHg, pO_2 95 mmHg, O_2 saturation 95%, Na 115 mEq/dL, glucose 156 mg/dL. What would be your next step in managing this patient?

Answer 9

The hyponatremia is the most pressing concern at this moment and should be corrected by having the surgeon stop all irrigating fluids and starting an infusion of 3% sodium chloride with the goal of correcting Na at a rate no greater than 0.5 mEq/hr. The hypertonic saline should be continued until the symptoms resolve or the serum sodium level reaches 120 mEq/dL, at which point I would switch the infusion to normal saline.

Question 10

You decide to keep the patient intubated and continue the 3% sodium chloride drip. The vital signs are stable and despite discontinuing all anesthetics the patient is unresponsive. What are you concerned about?

Answer 10

My concern would be that a cerebral vascular event or some metabolic disturbance has occurred. The stability of the vital signs argues against any cardiac etiology since hemodynamic instability would be expected.

Question 11

How would you manage this situation?

Answer 11

I would look at the vital signs to make sure the patient is not hypoxic, hypercarbic, hypotensive, or in a malignant arrhythmia. Next, I would recheck twitches (paralytic overdose), assess the eyes for pinpoint pupil (opioid overdose), and end tidal volatile anesthetic concentration to rule out any anesthetic-induced causes. I would also send an ABG and an electrolyte panel to look for potential hypo- or hyperglycemia, but especially to evaluate the serum sodium level. Finally, if none of these were the cause, a CT scan of the head might rule in or rule out any cerebral vascular event.

C. Postoperative Management

Central Pontine Myelinolysis

Question 1

A stat Na level in the PACU comes back at 128 mEq/dL. It was 115 mEq/dL 2 hours ago. What are your concerns?

Answer 1

The rapid rise in serum sodium is concerning, as it may result in the patient developing central pontine myelinolysis, a severe demyelinating condition of the brainstem. This state occurs in response to rapid increases in serum osmolality, indirectly measured using serum sodium levels.

Glycine Toxicity

Question 2

The patient recovers and is now awake in the recovery room. He reports blurry vision that progresses to blindness. What do you suspect is occurring?

Answer 2

In the setting of TURP surgery the onset of blindness is often associated with the use of glycine as an irrigating fluid. Glycine is structurally similar to GABA and is thus thought to stimulate inhibitory neural pathways, which result in the visual disturbances and may even result in transient blindness.

Question 3

How would you manage this situation?

Answer 3

The management of glycine-induced transient blindness is supportive and I would reassure the patient of the transient nature of the condition. Nonetheless, I would ask for an ophthalmologist to evaluate the patient for a more definitive diagnosis.

Question 4

Do you have any additional concerns with glycine toxicity?

Answer 4

Transient blindness is suggestive not only of excessive glycine absorption but also of elevated serum ammonia levels since glycine is metabolized into ammonia. The buildup of this by-product can result in altered mental status and even lead to coma until the body is able to adequately clear the metabolite. I would check a serum ammonia level and would want the patient to remain in a monitored setting in case he begins exhibiting mental status changes.

Oliguria

Question 5

The nurse reports that there has not been any urine output in the past hour. How would you evaluate the patient?

Answer 5

The normal urine output for an adult is 0.5 mL/kg/hr and anything less requires evaluation. Low urine output can be broken down into prerenal, intrarenal, and postrenal etiologies, and the evaluation should proceed systematically according to these categories. A prerenal etiology relates to a cardiac origin or to hypovolemia. Intrarenal etiology refers to actual kidney failure itself, whether from nephron damage or acute tubular necrosis. Postrenal causes are essentially due to physical obstructions to urine flow, whether from tumors, stones, or foreign bodies. The serum and urine electrolytes and creatinine should be checked to calculate the FeNa, or fractional excretion of sodium, which can help identify prerenal causes of low urine output. An ultrasound can be used to evaluate for kidney function as well as for any signs of urine flow obstruction. If there is a urinary catheter, it should be checked for kinks in the tubing, or it can be flushed to try to relieve any blockages.

Question 6

In addition to the low urine output the patient is tachycardic with a heart rate of 112 bpm and reports increasing bladder pressure. How would you manage this situation?

Answer 6

The findings are most likely indicative of catheter obstruction rather than any intrinsic renal condition. This patient underwent extensive tissue resection within the urethra and is likely forming clots that have obstructed the flow of urine. The urinary catheter should be flushed with saline to clear the obstruction and should then be placed on a continuous bladder irrigation. The continuous saline flow prevents the formation of potentially obstructing clots.

Suggested Readings

Atchabahian A, Gupta R, eds. *The Anesthesia Guide*. New York: McGraw Hill; 2013.

Barash PG, Cullen BF, Stoelting RK, Cahalan M, Stock CM, eds. *Clinical Anesthesia*. 6th ed. Philadelphia, PA: Lippincott Williams & Wilkins; 2009.

16 Pediatrics: Foreign Body Aspiration

Aimee Kakascik

Stem 2

An 18-month, 14 kg male is posted for diagnostic laryngoscopy, bronchoscopy, and foreign body removal. The parents noticed that he turned blue and became unresponsive while the family was eating popcorn and watching a movie. 911 was called and emergency service performed cardiopulmonary resuscitation (CPR). He arrived at the hospital ER after being unresponsive for 15 minutes. The child is currently somnolent with saturations of 93% on a nonrebreathable mask. His blood pressure is 90/54 mmHg, pulse 120 BPM, respirations 32. He has an 18-gauge intraosseous line.

A. Preoperative Evaluation

Respiratory

Question 1

How would you evaluate this patient's respiratory status?

Answer 1

I would perform a focused history and physical. From the history, assuming the parents are available, I would inquire about the sequence of events leading up to the child turning blue. Specifically, was the aspiration witnessed, and if so, what was the size and nature of the aspirated foreign material? I would also want to know specifically how long CPR had been performed and whether any emergency medicines such as epinephrine were administered. I would also want to know this patient's baseline respiratory status prior to the event, whether he had any symptoms of a respiratory infection, and any coexisting respiratory diseases such as asthma. From the physical exam, I would look at the child for increased work of breathing (retractions, nasal flaring, tripod posturing, drooling, and weakness). I would then examine the airway and auscultate the lungs looking for wheezing and decreased breath sounds on one side. A chest X-ray may indicate decreased lung volumes/atelectasis or hyperaeration of the ipsilateral affected side.

Question 2

What is your differential diagnosis for this patient?

Answer 2

My differential includes foreign body aspiration, esophageal foreign body, croup, reactive airway disease, anaphylactic reaction, epiglottitis, pneumonia, seizure, and cardiac anomaly/arrhythmia.

Question 3

How will you determine the correct diagnosis?

Answer 3

I will auscultate the chest. If there are decreased breath sounds on the right it is most likely a foreign body aspiration. Inspiratory and expiratory radiographic films should be obtained or lateral decubitus if for a small child. A mediastinal shift should occur toward the normal side when a foreign body is aspirated.

Vascular Access

Question 4

How do you place an intraosseous line?

Answer 4

To place an intraosseous line, I would prep the puncture site with a topical antiseptic, insert either an interosseous needle or a spinal needle into the proximal tibia two fingerbreadths distal to the tibial tuberosity, and advance it in a screwlike motion until a loss of resistance was obtained. The needle at this point should be firmly anchored in the bone. Finally, I would connect the infusion line and check for any extravasation of fluid.

Airway

Question 5

The child last ate popcorn 3 hours ago. Would you delay the surgery because of his full stomach?

Answer 5

No. While I am concerned about the increased risk for aspiration, the child is also in respiratory distress with a foreign body, which may migrate and reobstruct the airway. Further respiratory distress may ensue with irritation and damage from the aspirate.

Question 6

Would you give any premedication to the child?

Answer 6

Yes. I would give an anticholinergic to dry up airway secretions and to minimize the vagal response to bronchoscopy.

B. Intraoperative Management

Anesthesia

Question 1

Would you perform a rapid sequence induction on this patient because of the full stomach?

Answer 1

No. I would perform an inhalational induction and promote spontaneous ventilation in order to avoid further distal migration of the foreign body, which can lead to total airway obstruction or make retrieval technically challenging.

Question 2

How would you manage this case if the child aspirated shortly after your induction?

Answer 2

I would turn the child's head to the side, suction the oropharynx in a Trendelenburg position, intubate, suction the endotracheal tube, and then ventilate with 100% oxygen.

Question 3

Assuming the aspiration is now resolved and the ETT is removed at the start of the case, what is your plan for maintaining anesthesia?

Answer 3

I would promote spontaneous ventilation and maintain a deep plane of anesthesia with a TIVA technique during the rigid bronchoscopy by the ENT. I would avoid nitrous oxide as it reduces the inspired concentration of oxygen and increases lung volume from air entrapment in the affected lung.

Question 4

The procedure is proceeding well but the surgeon informs you that the popcorn kernel is too large to fit though the bronchoscope and she must remove it with the forceps and the bronchoscope together. She states that she needs the vocal cords to not move. Will you give succinycholine?

Answer 4

I will initially give this patient a propofol bolus to deepen the plane of anesthesia. I would avoid administering succinycholine to this child as it is not indicated for routine use in the pediatric population. If, after the propofol bolus, the surgeon still does not have the desired relaxation, then I would administer a small dose of rocuronium, as a last resort.

Question 5

The surgeon loses grip of the foreign body while trying to remove it. You are unable to ventilate the patient now. What can be done to improve ventilation?

Answer 5

The surgeon should try to remove the foreign body immediately. If she is unable to retrieve it, I would ask the surgeon to push the foreign body distally into the right main bronchus to relieve the total airway obstruction. If this was not successful, I would place the patient into the lateral or prone position in an effort to dislodge the object. Finally, if none of these interventions were successful, the next step would be to place this patient on cardiopulmonary bypass.

Emergence

Question 6

The kernel is successfully removed. The surgeon states that this was traumatic to the patient's airway and there is much swelling. What can you do to reduce the airway edema?

Answer 6

I would administer steroids (dexamethasone 0.5–1.5 mg/kg), humidified oxygen, and nebulized racemic epinephrine.

Question 7

Would you intubate the patient at the end of the procedure or allow the patient to wake up without an ETT?

Answer 7

It depends. I would discuss with the surgeon the extent of edema. I would then place a 3.5 cuffed ETT in the patient and measure the airway pressure at which he has an air leak (ideally between 25 and 30 mmHg). If the patient does not have a leak at this pressure, then most likely there is sufficient swelling to cause airway compromise. I would then leave the patient intubated overnight and allow the swelling to decrease.

Question 8

It has been 15 minutes and the patient has not awakened from the anesthesia. What could be the cause?

Answer 8

The possible causes for delayed awakening include hypoxia, hypercapnia, acidosis, hypotension, hypoglycemia, residual anesthesia, inadequate reversal of muscle relaxants, and possible neurological damage during the arrest.

C. Postoperative Management

Postoperative Stridor

Question 1

You decide to extubate the patient and take him to the recovery area. While in recovery the nurse calls you for a breathing treatment because the patient sounds "noisy." What could be the cause?

Answer 1

The child's airway could be obstructed from soft tissue relaxation, mucosal edema, or bronchospasm from airway irritation due to residual foreign body fragments.

Question 2

How would you assess the patient?

Answer 2

I would go immediately to the bedside and look at the patient's vital signs. I would also conduct a focused history and physical, reviewing what medications were given in the OR and in the PACU and asking the nurse if this occurred suddenly or gradually. I would also auscultate the lungs while assessing for increased work of breathing and level of consciousness.

Question 3

The patient has upper airway stridor. How will you treat this?

Answer 3

I will administer humidified oxygen, steroids, and nebulized racemic epinephrine while monitoring the vital signs, especially the EKG. If the patient has severe obstruction with unstable vital signs and depressed consciousness, I would reintubate with a smaller endotracheal tube and keep him ventilated overnight or until mucosal edema subsides.

Question 4

What is the mechanism of action of racemic epinephrine?

Answer 4

It stimulates α-receptors, resulting in vasoconstriction and secondary reduction in mucosal and submucosal edema.

Question 5

You gave racemic epinephrine an hour ago and now the patient is awake and alert with a room air saturation of 98%. The nurse asks you if the child can be discharged to the ward. What is your response?

Answer 5

No. I would not discharge the patient from recovery at this point, as it has been too soon after epinephrine administration and the patient could have "rebound" edema. Even though he has responded to the racemic epinephrine, he should be monitored for at least 3 hours after receiving the last dose to make sure "rebound" edema does not occur.

Postoperative Nausea

Question 6

The child vomited in recovery. How will you treat him?

Answer 6

I would go to the beside and ensure that the child's vital signs are stable. I would also check electrolytes and fluid status as hypoglycemia and hypovolemia can contribute to nausea. Assuming all of these were normal, I would administer a dose of a 5-HT3 antagonist, such as ondansetron, and also a steroid, such as dexamethasone (which may already have been given for airway edema).

Question 7

The mother says that "phenergan" was the only thing that helped her nausea after her Cesarean section and asks if her son can have it. What is your response?

Answer 7

I cannot give promethazine or "phenergan" to her child. There is a US box warning that respiratory fatalities have been reported in children under 2 years of age. Thus, the use of promethazine is contraindicated in this age group. In children 2 years of age and older, the lowest possible dose should be used and other drugs with respiratory depressant effects should be avoided.

Suggested Readings

American Heart Association. *PALS Provider Manual*. Minneapolis, MN: American Heart Association; 2006: 163–164. http://media.hsl.washington.edu/media/safranek/fpin/croup-guideline.pdf

Gregory GA, Andropoulos DB, eds. *Gregory's Pediatric Anesthesia*. 5th ed. Hoboken, NJ: Wiley-Blackwell; 2012: 368, 792–795.

US Food and Drug Administration. http://www.fda.gov/Safety/MedWatch/SafetyInformation/SafetyAlertsforHumanMedicalProducts/ucm152554.htm

17 Pediatrics: Tracheoesophageal Fistula Repair

Peggy Wingard

Stem 1

A 48-hour-old full-term infant male weighing 3 kg is brought to the OR for a type C tracheoesophageal fistula (TEF) repair.

History of present illness: The patient was delivered without complications. The mother of the patient had minimal prenatal care.

Past medical history: The patient was delivered via vaginal delivery.

Physical exam: Vital signs: HR 135 bpm, RR 30, BP 55/30 mmHg, SPO_2 98% on ½ L/min oxygen via nasal cannula (NC).

Lungs: Clear to auscultation bilaterally.

Cardiac: No murmurs were heard on heart exam.

X-rays: A blind pouch was noted on a lateral view, gas bubbles in the stomach were noted on chest/abdomen views.

Chest X-ray: No infiltrates seen.

Echocardiogram: Normal cardiac physiology with left-sided aorta arch.

EKG: Sinus tachycardia with T-wave inversions in leads V1–V4.

Labs: ABG pH 7.39, $PaCO_2$ 45 mmHg, PaO_2 85 mmHg, electrolytes are normal with glucose level of 50 mg/dL.

The neonate is brought to the OR with a 24 gauge IV and an A-line in place.

A. Preoperative Evaluation

Tracheoesophageal Fistula

Question 1

What is meant by a "type C" TEF?

Answer 1

A type C TEF has an esophageal atresia (ends blindly in the mediastinum at the level of T2 or T3) with a fistula connecting the distal esophageal pouch to the trachea.

There are five types of TEF, according to the classic Gross classification:

Type A—esophageal atresia with no connection to the trachea (8%)

Type B—esophageal atresia with a fistula connecting the proximal esophageal pouch to the trachea (<1%)

Type C—esophageal atresia with a fistula connecting the distal esophageal pouch to the trachea (75%)

Type D—fistulas connecting the proximal and distal esophageal pouches (2%)

Type E, the "H-type" fistula—intact esophagus with a fistula connecting to the trachea; there is no esophageal atresia (4%),

Type F—esophageal stenosis solely with no connection to the trachea

This child has the most common form of a TEF (Type C); more than 75% of all TEFs are of this type.

Question 2

How is a TEF diagnosed?

Answer 2

The diagnosis is made at birth when the nasogastric tube (NGT) is unable to be passed beyond 9–10 cm from the mouth and there is increased drooling or when the neonate develops episodes of coughing, choking, and/or cyanosis with the first feeding.

Question 3

What other congenital abnormalities are associated with TEFs?

Answer 3

Associated abnormalities can be remembered by the mnemonic VACTERL. When a child has three or more of the following abnormalities, he or she is considered to have VACTERL association.

V—vertebral/skeletal anomalies (10%)

A—anal canal defects, including anal atresia (14%)

C—cardiac anomalies, including ventricular septal defect, atrial septal defect, tetralogy of Fallot, right-sided aortic arch, and patent ductus arteriosus (30–50%)

TE—TEF

R—renal dysplasia, including malposition, hydronephrosis, and ureteral abnormalities (14%)

L—limb defects, including radial aplasia

Other associated anomalies include GI anomalies involving malrotation of the midgut and duodenal atresia.

Respiratory Status

Question 4

What measures can be taken to minimize aspiration preoperatively?

Answer 4

This patient should have a tube (usually a Replogle) placed into his blind-ending esophagus with continual suction and irrigation so that the chances of aspiration are minimized. Also, the head should be at a 30° head-up position and the patient kept NPO once the TEF is diagnosed.

Question 5

Would you insist on a gastrostomy tube placement prior to induction?

Answer 5

No. The current thinking is that gastrostomies are no longer done routinely unless there is concern for severe respiratory issues. The concern of having a gastrostomy in place is that by decompressing the stomach, gas from the trachea bypasses the lungs and exits through the stomach.

B. Intraoperative Management

Monitors

Question 1

What monitors would you use for this TEF repair?

Answer 1

I would use standard ASA monitors, including a pre- and postductal pulse oximeter, a preductal arterial line, and a precordial stethoscope.

Induction and Intubation

Question 2

What are your induction goals for this case?

Answer 2

My primary goal is to adequately ventilate the lungs without ventilating through the fistula, resulting in abdominal distention. Other goals include avoiding hemodynamic instability, aspiration, and maintaining normothermia.

Question 3

How would you secure the airway in this patient?

Answer 3

After performing an inhalational induction with oxygen and sevoflurane, I would place the ETT down the right mainstem (confirming with auscultation) with the bevel of the ETT facing forward and slowly withdraw the ETT until breath sounds become equal bilaterally. My goal is to have the ETT distal to the fistula and proximal to the carina. I would avoid muscle relaxation until the ETT was confirmed to be in the correct position.

Positioning

Question 4

If the patient desaturates during positioning at the start of the case, what is your differential diagnosis?

Answer 4

The ETT could have slipped into the right mainstem, preventing ventilation of the left lung. Alternatively, there could be increased gastric distention causing compromised ventilation. If the patient had a Fogarty catheter in place, I would be concerned that the catheter had slipped into the trachea, causing partial or total occlusion of the trachea. Other possibilities could include a kinked ETT, a disconnected ETT, or mucus and secretions occluding the ETT.

Question 5

If this desaturation occurred in the middle of the case, how would this change your differential diagnosis?

Answer 5

In addition to the causes previously mentioned, others include surgical manipulation of the (soft) trachea causing kinking or displacement of the ETT, surgical compression of vital structures in the mediastinum, and/or compression of the lung, resulting in atelectasis.

Question 6

How would you resolve the desaturation in either situations?

Answer 6

I would immediately place the child on 100% oxygen, reassess the other vital signs, confirm placement of the ETT by auscultation with the precordial stethoscope, and listen over the epigastric area for an air leak. I would also call for help, send off an ABG, and notify the surgeon. I would suction the ETT and manually ventilate the patient to assess for compliance as well as provide gentle positive pressure ventilation in the case of atelectasis.

Question 7

Can a tension pneumoperitoneum cause the desaturation? What is the mechanism?

Answer 7

Yes, it can. If there was increasing gastric distension, the stomach could rupture, leading to a pneumoperitoneum, which would impair ventilation.

C. Postoperative Care

Extubation

Question 1

Would you extubate this patient at the end of the case?

Answer 1

No. In addition to the increased risk for postoperative apnea in a child of less than 60 weeks' gestation, I am also concerned about the tension that would be placed at the anastomotic site if this patient were extubated and breathing spontaneously. Instead, I would prefer to have this patient sedated and relaxed until the anastomosis has had a chance to heal (at least 5 days) and would ensure adequate pain control.

Question 2

What postoperative pain management techniques would you use?

Answer 2

I would have this patient on a continuous fentanyl infusion of 0.5 to 2 mcg/kg/hr.

Complications of TEF Repair

Question 3

What are the early complications for this kind of surgical repair?

Answer 3

Early complications include anastomotic leaks and strictures. Some of the leaks will seal spontaneously and others may require surgical intervention. Strictures can occur at the site of the esophageal anastomosis or the fistula.

Question 4

What are the late complications for this kind of surgical repair?

Answer 4

Gastroesophageal reflux is the most common and significant long-standing problem after TEF or esophageal atresia repair. Other long-term issues include strictures, recurrent aspiration, pneumonia, recurrent lower and upper respiratory infections, reactive airway disease, feeding issues, and oral aversion. Decreased mucociliary clearance also occurs secondary to epithelial cells lacking cilia at the site of the TEF.

Esophageal dysmotility is associated with reduced intrinsic innervation. Tracheomalacia is significant in about 10% of patients and generally identified close to the site of the TEF. Abnormal pulmonary functions include abnormal expiratory flow rates, reduced lung volume, and airway hyperreactivity. There might be associated musculoskeletal malformations secondary to the thoracostomy, leading to winged scapula and chest wall asymmetry. Vocal cord paresis has also been reported.

Suggested Readings

Davis PJ, Cladis FP, Motoyama EK, eds. *Smith's Anesthesia for Infants and Children.* 8th ed. Philadelphia, PA: Mosby; 2011.

Gregory G, Andropoulos DB, eds. *Gregory's Pediatric Anesthesia.* 5th ed. Hoboken, NJ: Blackwell; 2012.

Yao FF, Artusio JF, eds. *Yao and Artusio's Anesthesiology: Problem-Oriented Patient Management.* 6th ed. Philadelphia, PA: Lippincott Williams & Wilkins; 2008.

18 Pediatrics: Pyloric Stenosis

Julio Olaya

Stem 2

A 2.9 kg male infant delivered 21 days ago at 40 weeks' gestation presents with a 48-hour history of nonbilious projectile vomiting. The child appears lethargic and weak on physical exam. There is a small palpable abdominal mass about 3 cm below the right costal margin with visible peristalsis. His vital signs are BP 55/36 mmHg, HR 157 bpm, RR 35, T 37°C. Hct = 56%. The patient has an older brother diagnosed with malignant hyperthermia (MH).

A. Preoperative Evaluation

Malignant Hyperthermia

Question 1

Do you need to send this patient to have a halothane caffeine contracture test (HCCT) to rule out malignant hyperthermia?

Answer 1

No, because this patient has a first-degree relative with a known diagnosis of MH. This alone places the patient at increased risk for developing an MH episode. Thus the child should be treated with full MH precautions.

Pyloric Stenosis

Question 2

What is your differential diagnosis for this child's presentation?

Answer 2

Highest on my differential list would be pyloric stenosis. This patient is presenting the classic signs associated with pyloric stenosis, such as male gender, projectile nonbilious vomiting, palpable olive mass with visible peristalsis, and an average age of onset in the range of 5 days to 5 months. Other differential diagnoses include achalasia of the esophagus, duodenal atresia, jejunal/ileal atresia, malrotation of the gut, intra-abdominal hernia, and Meckel's diverticulum.

Question 3

How would you confirm the diagnosis of pyloric stenosis?

Answer 3

A definitive diagnosis requires an abdominal ultrasound, but a thorough history and physical will reveal classic signs of a palpable mass, projectile vomiting, male gender, and laboratory data consistent with a hypokalemic, hypochloremic metabolic alkalosis.

Question 4

What electrolyte abnormalities would you expect in this patient?

Answer 4

I would expect to find a hypokalemic, hypochloremic metabolic alkalosis with a compensatory excretion of bicarbonate from the kidneys as well as a compensatory respiratory acidosis. If the electrolyte imbalance is not corrected and the patient continues to dehydrate, there will be a shift toward a metabolic acidosis.

Fluids

Question 5

How would you assess this patient's volume status?

Answer 5

I would perform a focused history and physical exam. From the history, I would inquire about the frequency and quantity of recent wet diapers, the volume and frequency of the projectile vomiting, and whether the patient has received any IV fluids thus far. From the physical, I would assess the vital signs, mucus membranes, presence of sunken fontanels, capillary refill, skin turgor, and mental status.

Question 6

Your resident suggests using lactated Ringer's for hydration. How do you respond?

Answer 6

Given the metabolic alkalosis, lactated Ringer's should be avoided since lactate is converted to bicarbonate, thereby worsening the acid–base imbalance. If the patient has a low urine output I would use normal saline until normal diuresis is established. Then I would switch to half normal saline, supplementing it with potassium and dextrose.

Question 7

How do you explain this patient's hematocrit value?

Answer 7

This child's elevated hematocrit value is most likely due to hemoconcentration as a result of the dehydration and frequent vomiting.

Question 8

The surgical resident tells you the GI obstruction is a surgical emergency and that the patient must be transferred to the OR immediately. How do you respond?

Answer 8

I would tell him that this is not a surgical emergency and that the patient needs to be adequately volume resuscitated and optimized before going to the OR.

B. Intraoperative Management

Malignant Hyperthermia

Question 1

How does the child's family history of MH affect your anesthetic management?

Answer 1

Given his family history of MH, I would avoid triggering agents like inhalational agents and succinylcholine. I would opt for a TIVA technique and have the MH cart in the room. I would also transduce an A-line and have proper resuscitation equipment in the room.

Monitoring

Question 2

Which monitors would you use intraoperatively?

Answer 2

I would use the standard ASA monitors (pulse oximetry, EKG, $EtCO_2$, BP cuff, and temperature probe).

Anesthesia and Induction

Question 3

How would you induce the patient?

Answer 3

Given the severe risk for aspiration, the stomach needs to be decompressed via either nasogastric (NG) or orogastric (OG) tube in the lateral, supine, and prone positions to remove as much of the gastric contents as possible. After pretreating with atropine (0.02 mg/kg IV) and decompressing the stomach with an OG tube, I would preoxygenate with 100% oxygen and perform a rapid sequence induction with cricoid pressure to minimize the risk of aspiration. My choice of induction agents are fentanyl, lidocaine, propofol, and rocuronium.

Pediatric Airway

Question 4

What are the key differences between the newborn and adult airways?

Answer 4

Newborns have narrow nasal passages, a large tongue, a long and pendulous epiglottis, and a funnel-shaped larynx. The position of the neonatal glottis is at the level of C3–C4, as opposed to C6 in adults. It is important to note that the narrowest portion in the neonate's airway is 1 cm below the vocal cords (at the level of the cricoid), whereas in adults it is at the level of the vocal cords.

Question 5

What size ETT would you use in this child?

Answer 5

I would use a 3.0 cuffed ETT for this child. In general, the ETT size for a full-term newborn is a 3.0 mm, at 6 months 3.5 mm, and at 1 year of age 4.0 mm. Once the patient is between the ages of 2 and 12 years, the following guide may be applied:

Tube length from tip to incisor teeth (cm) would be equal to 11 plus the age in years.

Tube Internal diameter (mm) = 4 + age / 4

Bronchospasm

Question 6

After intubating the patient you notice difficulty with ventilation. Your resident suggests placing the patient on sevoflurane in order to break the bronchospasm. What are you going to do?

Answer 6

I would not do this because this patient is susceptible to MH. Instead, I would begin by immediately switching to 100% oxygen, reassessing the other vital signs, deepening the TIVA anesthetic, checking the ETT position, administering a beta2 agonist like albuterol, and consider giving epinephrine if the symptoms do not improve.

C. Postoperative Management

Croup

Question 1

What are the primary postoperative concerns with this patient?

Answer 1

The primary concerns are continued risk of aspiration and pulmonary dysfunction, including apnea spells secondary to either metabolic alkalosis, hypothermia, or residual anesthesia. I would also be concerned about hypoglycemia from depletion of liver glycogen stores. Finally, postextubation "croup" is a potentially dangerous complication in this age group.

Question 2

How would you treat postextubation "croup" in this patient?

Answer 2

Immediate attention should be paid to a potential catastrophic postextubation laryngeal edema and management should be carried out by experienced pediatric anesthesiologists.

This includes the following:

Increased inspired oxygen concentration to around 50% to 60%, nebulized Vaponefrin therapy, humidification of inspired gases, and avoidance of excessive narcotics to avoid respiratory depression.

Steroids can be helpful and reintubation should be considered if signs of respiratory distress and hypoxia develop.

Postoperative Apnea

Question 3

Is this patient at increased risk for postoperative apnea?

Answer 3

Yes. Postoperative respiratory depression occurs commonly in patients with pyloric stenosis. The etiology is unclear but may be due to cerebrospinal fluid (CSF) alkalosis and intraoperative hyperventilation. In addition, infants up to 60 weeks postconceptual age are at increased risk for postoperative apnea. This patient is only 43 weeks.

Postoperative Hypoglycemia

Question 4

Two hours into the patient's PICU stay you notice that the patient has no dextrose in his IV fluid. Are you concerned?

Answer 4

Yes. Neonates after pylorotomy are at increased risk for postoperative hypoglycemia due to inadequate glycogen stores. Thus, I would immediately switch to dextrose-containing solutions and monitor the patient's blood sugar closely.

Suggested Readings

Hines RL, Marshall KE. *Stoelting's Anesthesia and Co-existing Disease*. Philadelphia, PA: Churchill Livingstone; 2008:599–600.

Kachko L, Simhi E, Freud E, Dlugy E, Katz J. Impact of spinal anesthesia for open pyloromyotomy on operating room time. *J Pediatr Surg*. 2009;44(10):1942–1946.

Wolfson AB, Cloutier RL, Hendey GW, Ling LJ, Schaider JJ, Rosen CL, eds. *Harwood-Nuss' Clinical Practice of Emergency Medicine Clinical Practice of Emergency Medicine*. Philadelphia, PA: Wolters Kluver; 2015: 1310.

19 Pediatrics: Congenital Diaphragmatic Hernia

Peggy Wingard

Stem 1

A 7-day-old, preterm male weighting 2.5 kg is brought to the OR for repair of a left-sided congenital diaphragmatic hernia (CDH).

Past medical history: The child was intubated with a 2.5 ETT shortly after birth and placed on low-pressure ventilation for respiratory distress and cyanosis. Abdominal ultrasound confirmed the CDH. No other congenital malformations were noted.

Physical exam: Vital signs BP 50/25 mmHg, RR 60, HR 148 bpm, T 38°C.

Lungs—diminished breath sounds in the right chest, bowel sounds present in the left chest.

Cardiac—no murmurs noted but heart sounds are slightly displaced to the right.

Abdomen—scaphoid appearance.

Labs: ABG: pH 7.26, $PaCO_2$ = 55 mmHg, PaO_2 = 80 on 30% FiO_2, Hb = 16 g/dL, Hct 49%.

Chest X-rays: Presence of gas-filled loops of bowel in the left hemi-diaphragm.

The neonate is brought to the OR with a 24 gauge IV and an A-line.

A. Preoperative Evaluation

Emergent or Nonemergent Surgery

Question 1

Is this an emergent surgery? Why or why not?

Answer 1

Historically, this kind of procedure was considered to be an emergency, but current thinking is that the patient must first be medically managed prior to surgery. Medical management of this patient includes stabilizing the cardiorespiratory function by improving oxygenation to have a preductal oxygen saturation >90%, correcting acidosis, reduction of right-to-left (R → L) shunt, and increasing pulmonary perfusion (utilizing the least aggressive ventilation possible).

Respiratory and Circulatory

Question 2

Explain the physical exam findings associated with CDH.

Answer 2

The physical exam findings I would expect in a child with a CDH include a barrel chest, scaphoid abdomen, bowel sounds on chest auscultation, heart sounds displaced to the right because of the abdominal contents, respiratory distress, and hypoxemia.

Question 3

Why do patients with CDH develop respiratory distress and cyanosis?

Answer 3

Cyanosis results from (1) atelectasis from the compression of the abdominal contents into the developed lung; (2) pulmonary hypoplasia from the pressure of the herniated abdominal contents, resulting in decreased number of alveoli and bronchial generations with medial hyperplasia of pulmonary arterioles; and (3) persistent pulmonary hypertension causing increased R → L shunting through a patent foramen ovale and patent ductus arteriosus.

Question 4

What factors promote R → L shunting in neonates with CDH?

Answer 4

The most common factor is pulmonary hypertension, as increased pulmonary vascular resistance (PVR) promotes deoxygenated blood to be shunted through a patent foramen ovale or a patent ductus arteriosus. Other causes are an imbalance in the production, release, and levels of vasoconstrictors (leukotrienes C4, D4, thromboxane A2, platelet-activating factor) and vasodilators (nitric oxide [NO], prostacyclin).

Question 5

How would you treat this patient's pulmonary hypertension?

Answer 5

I would want to avoid situations that increase PVR, such as hypoxia and acidosis. I would have this patient sedated (to minimize stress-induced catecholamine secretion) and paralyzed (to reduce oxygen consumption) and avoid ventilating with 100% oxygen, as this will worsen pulmonary hypertension. Other maneuvers include administering NO (a selective pulmonary vasodilator that reduces PVR), high-frequency oscillatory ventilation (HFOV) (which improves ventilation while reducing barotrauma), and addition of prostaglandins E1 or D2. Extracorporeal membrane oxygenation (ECMO) could also be used in cases where conventional ventilatory maneuvers and HFOV have not worked and there is persistent preductal hypoxemia.

Question 6

What is the role of permissive hypercapnia in this child?

Answer 6

It is a technique that is thought to improve the overall survival of neonates with CHD. Small tidal volume and higher levels of PEEP are used to keep the airways open and allow a rise in PCO_2 (60 mmHg). The larger tidal volume needed to maintain normocarbia can cause volutrauma, inducing an inflammatory reaction and release of vasoactive mediators that lead to vasoconstriction and further lung injury (ultimately leading to ARDS). But I do need to be mindful that hypercarbia may worsen PVR.

Question 7

What is the mechanism of action of nitric oxide?

Answer 7

NO causes stimulation of cyclic guanylate cyclase, which increases cyclic guanosine monophosphate (GMP). Cyclic GMP activates protein kinases that cause relaxation of vascular smooth muscle.

B. Intraoperative Management

Monitors

Question 1

How are you going to monitor this neonate? If you had a central line, where would you place it? Why?

Answer 1

In addition to the standard ASA monitors and the A-line that is already in place, I would place preductal and postductal saturation monitors. I would place an umbilical central line in this specific patient for several reasons: monitoring of volume status, administration of inotropic agents, administration of blood if needed, and access for total parenteral nutrition (TPN). I would avoid lower extremity central-line placement due to inferior vena cava compression with reduction of the hernia. I would want to reserve the neonate's neck veins for possible ECMO therapy. Urine output would be measured with a Foley catheter.

Induction, Intubation, and Maintenance

Question 2

If this patient was not already intubated, how would you secure the airway in this child?

Answer 2

I would perform an inhalational induction, maintaining spontaneous ventilation, with oxygen and sevoflurane. I would avoid using positive pressure ventilation, which will further cause respiratory compromise.

Question 3

What agents would you use for maintenance? Can you use nitrous oxide (N_2O)?

Answer 3

Provided that the neonate is stable, I would use a combination of O_2/air to maintain oxygen saturation in the low to mid 90s, sevoflurane, fentanyl, and vecuronium. I would use low concentrations of sevoflurane because I am concerned that while these agents produce pulmonary vasodilation and decrease hypoxic pulmonary vasoconstriction (HPV), their effects on SVR are greater than their effects on PVR and may worsen the R → L shunt. I would not use N_2O for several reasons. I do not want N_2O to diffuse into the abdominal viscera, causing additional respiratory compromise and potentially strangulating the herniated bowels.

Ventilation

Question 4

What are your goals for ventilation? How are you going to achieve them?

Answer 4

My goals are to avoid barotrauma and provide adequate oxygenation. I would accomplish this by ensuring the airway measurements do not exceed 25–30 cm H_2O, a PEEP of 5 to 7 cm H_2O, oxygen saturation of 90% to 95%, and permissive hypercarbia as tolerated with a pH >7.25.

Question 5

Will you use 100% FiO_2 in this patient if you are worried about hypoxia?

Answer 5

No. In addition to the risk of the child developing retinopathy of prematurity (ROP), which is seen in patients younger than 44 weeks' gestation, I am concerned that 100% oxygen will worsen oxygenation and ventilation as it will recruit additional blood flow to an already less compliant lung and worsen pulmonary hypertension. I would only use 100% oxygen to reverse any acute periods of desaturation and hypoxia.

Decompensation

Question 6

One hour into the procedure, the patient's saturation drops to 80% and the blood pressure reads 40/20 mmHg. What do you think is happening?

Answer 6

At the top of my differential list is a pneumothorax in the contralateral lung. Other possibilities include severe pulmonary hypertension, compression of great vessels, acute blood loss, hypovolemia, hypothermia, or allergic reaction to a drug administered.

Question 7

How will you manage this situation?

Answer 7

I would immediately look at the other vital signs and make sure the patient is not in a malignant arrhythmia. I would open the fluids and place the patient on 100% oxygen temporarily while I probe for causes. I would inform the surgeon and auscultate the lungs to assess if a pneumothorax has occurred. If it has, a needle decompression should be carried out immediately and a chest tube placed by the surgeon. I would also avoid hyperventilation, to prevent air leak into the pneumothorax.

Question 8

(Examiner interrupts) It's not a pneumothorax. What else are you going to do?

Answer 8

I would then rule out reversible causes. I would instruct the surgeon to relieve compression on the great vessels if they were being surgically compressed. If this were caused by R → L shunting secondary to elevated pulmonary hypertension, I would expect a higher pulse oximeter reading on my preductal pulse oximeter than on the postductal pulse oximeter. I would take steps to reduce PVR (NO, hyperventilation) and increase SVR.

Question 9

How would hypothermia affect this patient?

Answer 9

Hypothermia causes an increase in PVR, which can lead to an increased R → L shunt though the patent ductus arteriosus (PDA) or patent foramen ovale (PFO).

Fluids

Question 10

Would you give glucose-containing solution during this procedure?

Answer 10

Yes. Neonates have decreased glycogen stores and are prone to developing hypoglycemia. Maintenance fluids would consist of D5/0.2% NaCl or D5/0.45% NaCl at 4 cc/kg/hr. Third space losses would be replaced with LR or 0.9% NaCl at 8 cc/kg/hr. Blood loss is replaced in a 1:3 ratio of blood/LR and a 1:1 ratio of blood/5% albumin. ABGs, vital signs, and CVP would guide further fluid replacement.

Question 11

Surgery is now completed. During skin closure the patient's BP drops again. What are you going to do?

Answer 11

This is most likely due to inferior vena cava compression, resulting in decreased cardiac output from diminished venous return. This compression will have to be relieved by opening the abdominal cavity and covering the abdominal defect temporarily with a Silastic patch.

C. Postoperative Care

Extubation

Question 1

Are you going to extubate this patient at the end of surgery?

Answer 1

No. I would leave this patient intubated and maintained on fentanyl and vecuronium infusions postoperatively in the neonatal intensive care unit (NICU). These patients are at high risk of various degrees of postoperative pulmonary dysfunction and I expect that the child will further decompensate after a brief honeymoon period.

Decompensation

Question 2

The child begins to desaturate after 6 hours in the NICU. What will you do?

Answer 2

I would go by the bedside and ensure that the other vital signs are stable. I would then listen to the lungs to make sure that a tension pneumothorax has not occurred, obtain an ABG, and assess for pulmonary hypertension.

Question 3

Would you place this patient on HFOV? ECMO?

Answer 3

If this neonate did not respond to maneuvers such as 100% oxygen, and hyperventilation from a conventional ventilator, I would place this patient on HFOV. If this ventilatory strategy did not work and pharmacological intervention did not improve the status, I would consider ECMO.

Question 4

What is ECMO? What are the advantages and disadvantages of ECMO?

Answer 4

It is a strategy to improve oxygenation/ventilation and myocardial dysfunction. It can be done via venovenous or venoarterial bypass. Venovenous bypass has a double-lumen catheter through the internal jugular (IJ) vein. Blood is removed from and infused into the RA through separate ports. Venoarterial bypass has the RA cannulated through the IJ vein where blood passively flows by gravity into the ECMO circuit, pumped into a member oxygenator and returned back to the patient through the right common carotid artery into the ascending aorta.

Advantages include elimination or significant reduction of R → L shunting through the PDA or PFO and reduction of right ventricular workload (decreased pulmonary blood flow and pressure), pulmonary vasoconstriction (secondary to correction of hypoxia and acidosis by ECMO), and incidence of bronchopulmonary dysplasia (FiO_2 requirements and airway pressure are decreased by ECMO).

Disadvantages include the need for anticoagulation, increased bleeding potential at the surgical and chest tube insertion sites, intracranial hemorrhage, and sepsis.

Question 5

Are there criteria for going on ECMO?

Answer 5

Yes, the criteria are $P(A\text{-}a)O_2$ >600 mmHg for more than 6–8 hours, O_2 index of 51 for 5 hours. O_2 index = $FiO_2 \times$ mean airway pressure/PaO_2, gestational age ≥34 weeks, weight ≥2 kg, and the presence of a reversible disease process.

Outcomes

Question 6

What are some of the long-term outcomes for these patients?

Answer 6

These patients may go on to develop reactive airway disease, obstructive lung disease requiring usage of bronchodilators and inhaled steroids, GERD, chest wall deformities, and scoliosis.

Suggested Readings

Davis PJ, Cladis FP, Motoyama EK, eds. *Smith's Anesthesia for Infants and Children.* 8th ed. Philadelphia, PA: Mosby; 2011.

Gregory G, Andropoulos DB, eds. *Gregory's Pediatric Anesthesia.* 5th ed. Hoboken, NJ: Blackwell; 2012.

Yao FF, Artusio JF, eds. *Yao and Artusio's Anesthesiology: Problem-Oriented Patient Management.* 6th ed. Philadelphia, PA: Lippincott Williams & Wilkins; 2008.

20 Pediatrics: Epiglottitis

Julio Olaya

Stem 2

A 2-year-old African American boy is brought to the ER for respiratory distress. The child is excessively drooling and leaning forward "to catch his breath." There are substernal retractions along with stridorous respirations. He is complaining of a sore throat. Vital signs are BP 101/80 mmHg, RR 33, HR 130 BPM, O_2 saturation 98% on 2 L oxygen, T 40°C.

A. Preoperative Evaluation

Diagnosis

Question 1

What is the most likely diagnosis in this patient?

Answer 1

This patient most likely has acute epiglottitis secondary to an infectious process. Epiglottitis is often bacterial in origin, and the most common causative agent is *Haemophilus* influenza type B.

Question 2

What are the clinical signs and symptoms of acute epiglottitis?

Answer 2

This condition usually begins with complaints of severe sore throat associated with dysphagia and muffled voice. The symptoms rapidly progress and typical pathognomonic signs of dyspnea, drooling, dysphagia, and dysphonia (i.e., the four Ds) manifest.

The illness presents acutely in otherwise healthy children between 2 and 5 years of age, with fever as high as 40°C (104°F). In a matter of a few hours the epiglottic inflammation evolves and the child becomes dyspneic. The child usually leans forward and excessive salivation is characteristic, as swallowing is difficult. The patient appears anxious and toxic with heavy concentration on breathing.

Question 3

Should you wait for culture studies to come back to definitively diagnose epiglottitis?

Answer 3

No. Acute epiglottitis is considered an emergency and thus a clinical diagnosis is often sufficient to transfer the patient to the OR for an emergent intubation. If an X-ray had already been completed, it would most likely show a "thumb print" sign on a lateral view.

Volume Status

Question 4

Are you concerned about the child's volume status? How would you assess the degree of dehydration?

Answer 4

Yes, I am concerned about his volume status. I would assess his volume status through a focused history from his parents and physical examination focusing on skin turgor, capillary refill, heart rate, blood pressure, and mental status.

Question 5

Would you place an IV in this patient before taking him to the OR?

Answer 5

No. The placement of an IV in an uncontrolled setting can precipitate a life-threatening episode of laryngospasm.

Selection of Anesthetic Technique

Question 6

The father of the patient asks you if you really need to give his child a full-blown general anesthetic (GA) for the intubation. How will you respond?

Answer 6

I would tell the father that a GA is absolutely necessary and that is has many benefits. First, it allows the surgeon to look at the area of the swelling, which would be very uncomfortable for an awake patient. Second, GA would prevent the child from being aware of what is being done to him. Third, GA allows us to maintain a secure airway, deliver oxygen continuously to the patient, and prevent the development of life-threatening hypoxia.

Question 7

How would you transfer this patient to the OR?

Answer 7

Timing is crucial. Once the diagnosis is made, the child is transported with his parents and a physician with proficiency in airway management (including an ENT surgeon) and emergency airway equipment (including a cricothyrotomy kit). I would avoid any kind of upsetting maneuvers, like trying to start an IV or separating the child from his parents, since crying can potentially trigger respiratory distress and airway obstruction. Nasal prongs or face tent oxygen should be provided and pulse oximetry should be used. Once in the OR, I would have the difficult-intubation cart available and an ENT surgeon on standby.

B. Intraoperative Management

Airway

Question 1

How are you going to secure the airway in this patient?

Answer 1

I would perform an inhalational induction with sevoflurane and oxygen with the child on a parent's lap in the OR. Once the patient became drowsy, I would transfer him sitting up onto the OR table and ask the parent to be escorted from the OR. Once a deep plane of anesthesia has been achieved, an intravenous line is placed and a careful direct laryngoscopy is performed. I would consider placing an ETT 0.5–1.0 mm smaller than the size I normally use.

Question 2

Your colleague suggests a rapid sequence induction because the NPO status is unclear. What will you say to him?

Answer 2

I would tell my colleague that a slow inhalational induction is the technique of choice because a rapid sequence induction might predispose the patient to severe hypoxia and hypoventilation if intubation is not achieved expeditiously. Once an IV has been established, I would give metoclopramide as a premedication prior to direct laryngoscopy, to minimize the chance of aspiration. In terms of NPO status, although it is possible that the patient has not fasted for 8 hours as he normally would had this been an elective case, children with epiglottitis often have difficulty in swallowing secondarily to the pain and discomfort. Thus it is unlikely that the patient has a full stomach, and even if it is it would not alter my management at this time.

Question 3

How about an awake intubation?

Answer 3

No, I would not perform an awake intubation because the risk of losing the airway is very high due to possible adenoidal bleeding, trauma, agitation, laryngospasm, and difficult visualization.

Question 4

After several intubation attempts, you are still unable to secure the airway. Mask ventilation is becoming progressively more difficult and his saturation is falling. What do you do?

Answer 4

I would call for help if I haven't already done so and employ jet ventilation to restore the child's saturation. In addition, I would reposition the patient's airway, switch to a different blade, downgrade the size of the ETT, and prepare for another direct laryngoscopy attempt while alerting the ENT surgeon for a possible surgical airway. My attempts to secure the airway using another airway device such as an LMA may be limited because of swelling of the epiglottis, which could lead to further airway obstruction. Thus, in the absence of endotracheal intubation, with further patient deterioration, I would want to proceed immediately with a surgical airway if jet ventilation fails.

C. Postoperative Management

Extubation

Question 1

Let's assume you had been able to intubate this patient on your first try. How long would you keep this patient intubated?

Answer 1

Usually, it is possible to extubate these patients within 24 to 48 hours.

Question 2

What will be your criteria to extubate this child?

Answer 2

My criteria would be a return of normal body temperature after appropriate antibiotic therapy with either cefazolin, ampicillin with sulbactam, ceftriaxone, or clindamycin; an increased leak around the endotracheal tube; and a decrease in erythema and edema.

Question 3

Would you keep this patient sedated while intubated?

Answer 3

Yes. It is important to minimize patient movement and accidental self-extubation.

Question 4

Is it necessary to admit this patient to the PICU?

Answer 4

Yes, it is necessary. This will allow for close supervision of the patient's vital signs, correction of fluid deficits, and adjustments to the ventilator settings.

Question 5

After 48 hours you decide to extubate the patient. Describe your technique.

Answer 5

First, I would ensure that the patient is afebrile with a positive leak test around the ETT. Next, I would transfer the patient to the OR, have ENT on standby with the neck prepped and draped, and induce general anesthesia to allow confirmation of resolution of the airway edema by direct visual inspection. Assuming the edema had resolved, I would extubate and continue to monitor him closely in the PACU.

Suggested Readings

Bass JW, Steele RW, Wiebe RA. Acute epiglottitis: a surgical emergency. *JAMA*. 1974;229(6):671–675.

DeSoto H. Epiglottitis and croup in airway obstruction in children. *Anesthesiol Clin*. 1998; 16(4):853–868.

21 Pediatrics: Patent Ductus Arteriosus

Peggy Wingard

Stem 1

A 30-week-old 1.3 kg male neonate, now 6 days old, presents for repair of a patent ductus arteriosus (PDA).

Past medical history: The patient was not treated medically for closure of his PDA. Surfactant was administered. The child was intubated shortly after birth with saturations maintained in the mid-80s; he is currently on pressure control ventilation but initially was on HFOV.

Physical exam: Vital signs: BP 45/20 mmHg, HR 178 bpm, RR 40, saturation 87% on 100% O_2.

Lungs—intubated with 3.0 ETT, taped at 8.5 cm at the lips.

Cardiac—S3 present, continuous systolic and diastolic murmur best heard at the left upper sternal border.

Head CT: Small intraventricular hemorrhage (IVH), grade 2.

Echocardiogram: PDA of moderate size is present.

Labs: Hgb 11 g/dL, Hct 33%, glucose 60 mg/dL.

The neonate is brought to the OR with two peripheral IVs in place.

A. Preoperative Evaluation

Prematurity

Question 1

What are some concerns with a premature neonate?

Answer 1

Besides his PDA and cardiac problems, such as shunt reversal, I am concerned about his pulmonary status (compliance, degree of pulmonary hypertension, if any), ventilator settings, signs of infection, necrotizing enterocolitis, and electrolyte imbalances, including hypo- or hyperglycemia. I am also concerned about hypocalcemia, temperature instability, anemia, IVH, and retinopathy of prematurity. In addition, status of TPN and IV access, status of renal and hepatic function (as little as 1 week on parenteral nutrition can cause organ toxicity), and whether the patient has been on chronic steroids that may require steroid coverage in the OR are of concern.

Question 2

Your resident asks why the patient can't receive medical treatment for the PDA closure with indomethacin in place of surgery. How do you respond?

Answer 2

Indomethacin is a nonselective cyclo-oxygenase inhibitor that decreases prostaglandin E1 levels and could cause increased intraventricular bleeding in this patient, who has already suffered a grade 2 IVH. Thus, indomethacin may not be a viable option. Additionally, perhaps the PDA is too large to be closed medically or a trial of indomethacin was administered and the patient did not respond.

Question 3

Are there any contraindications for using indomethacin in this setting?

Answer 3

Yes, the contraindications are intracranial hemorrhage (secondary to platelet dysfunction), renal dysfunction, and hyperbilirubinemia. Adverse effects of indomethacin include decreased mesenteric, renal, and cerebral blood flow.

Necrotizing Enterocolitis (NEC)

Question 4

Is this neonate at risk for developing NEC? Why?

Answer 4

Yes, he is, because with a PDA (especially large ones), blood is shunted away from the systemic circulation and toward the pulmonary circulation, resulting in decreased abdominal organ perfusion. Since the gut is one of the first organs to be deprived of blood, the child is at risk of developing NEC.

PDA

Question 5

How else can you make the diagnosis of PDA besides the characteristic murmur?

Answer 5

During evaluation of the neonate I would look for bounding pulses, widened pulse pressure, CHF manifested by intercostal retractions, decreased breath sounds, rales, and an S3 sound. Increasing respiratory failure with PaO_2 decreases and $PaCO_2$ increases require ventilatory support. An echocardiogram will confirm the presence of a PDA.

B. Intraoperative Management

Question 1

What monitoring would you use for this neonate? Does the presence of a PDA affect your choice of where to place the monitors?

Answer 1

I would use the standard ASA monitors (pulse oximeter, BP cuff, EKG, $EtCO_2$, and temperature probe [rectal]), a Foley catheter to measure urine output, and a central line if I do not have two well-running PIVs. I would also have an A-line placed in the right upper extremity since clamping of the left subclavian artery may become necessary should the PDA be torn during the procedure. I would place the pulse oximeters in the right hand and lower limb to measure both preductal and postductal readings.

Maintenance

Question 2

Would you use inhalational agents for maintenance?

Answer 2

Inhalation agents, such as sevoflurane, can be used because they are cheap and easily titratable. However, they can cause a decrease in SVR with resulting hypotension. Thus, my first choice would be a high-dose fentanyl (30–50 mcg/kg) technique.

Question 3

What is your target oxygen saturation in this patient? Why?

Answer 3

My target oxygen saturation in this patient is between 87% and 95% because this patient is at risk for retinopathy of prematurity. The child's risk factors are (1) prematurity (<32 weeks' gestation), (2) mechanical ventilation, (3) respiratory distress, (4) hypoxia, and (5) possible acidosis.

Complications

Question 4

Midway through the case, the blood pressure suddenly drops and the patient begins to desaturate. What is your differential diagnosis?

Answer 4

My differential would be as follows:

Airway causes: Disconnected ETT, kinked or occluded circuit or ETT

Hemodynamic causes: Malignant arrhythmia, PE

Surgical causes: Hemorrhage secondary to tearing of the ductus, ligation of descending aorta or pulmonary artery, lung retraction, pneumothorax

Question 5

What will you do?

Answer 5

I would quickly evaluate the patient by looking at the vital signs, EKG, and $EtCO_2$; examining the ETT and listening for bilateral breath sounds; looking over the drapes for bleeding; and looking at the suction canisters as well as sponges and lap pads.

Postligation

Question 6

What is the vital sign most affected immediately after ligation of the PDA?

Answer 6

Ligation of the PDA may cause systemic hypertension, resulting in an increased left ventricular afterload or elevated cerebral perfusion pressure. If the blood pressure rise is not transient, I would administer a vasodilator drug such as nitroprusside or nitroglycerin If the increased left ventricular afterload causes severe dysfunction of the left ventricle, I would place the patient on an inotropic agent such as dopamine.

C. Postoperative Care

Postoperative Issues

Question 1

Should this patient be on antibiotics postoperatively? For how long?

Answer 1

For 6 months following artificial closure this neonate should receive subacute bacterial endocarditis (SBE) prophylaxis when undergoing any surgical procedures.

Question 2

Would you extubate this neonate if everything went well intraoperatively?

Answer 2

No, I would not extubate this patient. This patient had a relatively large shunt and is a 31-week premie who initially was on HFOV and came to the OR on a pressure control ventilator. Additionally, he was placed on dopamine in the OR and has a relatively large incision that may impair ventilation postoperatively due to pain. This patient may benefit from mechanical ventilation for a significant time after surgery.

Had this had been a healthy, asymptomatic infant and the procedure went well, I would have considered extubating the neonate in the OR.

PDA Physiology

Question 3

Under what circumstances would you want a PDA to maintain its patency?

Answer 3

When there is an undiagnosed cardiac condition that has ductal-dependent system circulation such as hypoplastic left heart syndrome, aortic valve stenosis, interrupted aortic arch, or coarctation of the aorta. The PDA should be reopened with prostaglandin E1 (0.05–0.1 mcg/kg/min) until the definitive surgical procedure is performed.

Complications

Question 4

What are some complications that are associated postoperatively with PDA ligation?

Answer 4

Depending on the surgical approach, some complications include recurrent laryngeal nerve paralysis and chest wall deformities such as cosmetic defects, scoliosis, and rib fusion. These deformities may be minimized by a percutaneously inserted coil or an occlusion device or by doing the procedure via video-assisted thoracoscopic surgery (VATS). Another complication to avoid is retinopathy of prematurity.

Suggested Readings

Davis PJ, Cladis FP, Motoyama EK, eds. *Smith's Anesthesia for Infants and Children*. 8th ed. Philadelphia, PA: Mosby; 2011.

Gregory G, Andropoulos DB, eds. *Gregory's Pediatric Anesthesia*. 5th ed. Hoboken, NJ: Blackwell; 2012.

Hines RL, Marschall KE, eds. *Stoelting's Anesthesia and Co-Existing Disease*. 5th ed. Philadelphia, PA: Saunders Elsevier; 2008.

Litman R. *Pediatric Anesthesia, The Requisites in Anesthesiology*. Philadelphia, PA: Mosby; 2004.

22 Pediatrics: Tetralogy of Fallot

Kseniya Khmara and Ruchir Gupta

Stem 2

A 6-month-old female is scheduled for a tetralogy of Fallot repair. The patient has a history of progressively worsening cyanotic episodes since birth. Vital signs are BP 60/30 mmHg, HR 110 bpm, RR 30, O_2 saturation 94% on RA. Hct = 55%.

A. Preoperative Evaluation

Definition

Question 1

What is tetralogy of Fallot?

Answer 1

Tetralogy of Fallot is a cyanotic heart defect characterized by a constellation of four major anomalies: pulmonic stenosis, ventricular septal defect (VSD), overriding aorta, and right ventricular hypertrophy. Blood is shunted from the right side of the heart to the left, bypassing the pulmonary circulation.

Question 2

What is the main difference between cyanotic and acyanotic cardiac lesions?

Answer 2

In cyanotic cardiac lesions, a fraction of deoxygenated blood from the right side of the heart bypasses the lungs and is shunted into the systemic circulation. Thus, blood ejected from the left ventricle is an admixture of oxygenated and deoxygenated blood. In acyanotic cardiac lesions, oxygenated blood from the left side of the heart is shunted over into the pulmonary circulation. Thus blood that is ejected from the left ventricle into the systemic circulation remains purely oxygenated.

Tet Spells

Question 3

The parents mention that the patient's "Tet spells" have been progressively getting worse. How does a "Tet spell" happen?

Answer 3

"Tet spells" are hypercyanotic attacks that occur when there is a relative increase in right-sided heart pressures that further promote right-to-left intracardiac shunting of deoxygenated blood. An elevated right-sided heart pressure can be caused by an increase in pulmonary vascular resistance, right ventricular outflow obstruction (usually due to a stenotic pulmonic valve), and/or a decrease in systemic vascular resistance. Often, normal activities such as crying, feeding, defecating, and exercise can induce a "Tet spell."

Question 4

If this child were to develop a "Tet spell" in the holding area, how would you manage the situation without an IV?

Answer 4

First, I would call for help and have emergency medications on standby. Next, I would reassess the vital signs while placing the baby on the parent's shoulder with the infant's knees tucked up underneath. This reduces systemic venous return and increases SVR.

Antibiotic Prophylaxis

Question 5

Do you plan on administering antibiotic prophylaxis for infective endocarditis? Which antibiotic would you administer if there is an IV in place?

Answer 5

Yes. I would administer amoxicillin 50 mg/kg IV.

Question 6

If the child has allergies to penicillin, what is your backup antibiotic prophylaxis for infective endocarditis treatment?

Answer 6

Clindamycin 20 mg/kg IV.

Question 7

What cardiac conditions require infective endocarditis antibiotic prophylaxis?

Answer 7

- Prosthetic cardiac valve or prosthetic material used for cardiac valve repair
- History of infective endocarditis
- Unrepaired cyanotic congenital heart defect (CHD) (including palliative shunts and conduits)
- For the first 6 months after completely repairing a congenital heart defect with prosthetic material or device

- Repaired CHD with residual defects at the site or adjacent to the site of a prosthetic patch or prosthetic device
- Valvulopathy after cardiac transplantation

B. Intraoperative Management

Induction

Question 1

What are your hemodynamic goals in this patient?

Answer 1

The hemodynamic goals in this patient are to avoid conditions that will lower the SVR and/or increase the PVR. Any deviation from baseline parameters will induce a right-to-left shunting with the development of hypoxemia.

Question 2

How are you going to induce this patient?

Answer 2

After preoxygenating with 100% oxygen, I would perform a smooth IV induction with ketamine (1–2 mg/kg), fentanyl, and rocuronium. The benefit of using ketamine in this child is that it will maintain or increase the SVR, thereby avoiding a "Tet spell."

Question 3

Would you use succinylcholine in this patient?

Answer 3

No. I want to avoid using succinylcholine for two reasons:

1. It is not indicated for routine use in the pediatric population because of the increased risk for malignant hyperthermia as well as hyperkalemic cardiac arrest secondary to undiagnosed myopathy.
2. Succinylcholine is associated with histamine release, which can decrease the SVR and promote further right-to-left shunting of blood.

Onset Time of Agents

Question 4

Your resident asks if a mask induction technique with sevoflurane is preferred for a child with TOF. How do you respond?

Answer 4

No. A mask induction technique is not ideal in this setting as sevoflurane can reduce the SVR in this patient and promote right-to-left shunting.

Question 5

How does the presence of a shunt affect the onset time of your IV induction agents in a child with TOF?

Answer 5

The presence of a baseline right-to-left shunt can speed up the onset time of IV agents since more blood is diverted into the systemic circulation and to end-target vessel-rich organs.

Maintenance

Question 6

What agents would you use for maintenance?

Answer 6

I would want to use a mixture of nitrous oxide, oxygen, and ketamine. While nitrous oxide is associated with an increase in PVR, these effects are outweighed by the beneficial effect on SVR (no change or modest increase). I would limit the inspired concentration on nitrous to 50%, to provide adequate FiO_2 and minimize hypoxia, which can lead to an increase in PVR.

Question 7

What are the advantages and disadvantages of nitrous oxide for this patient?

Answer 7

The benefit of nitrous oxide is that is maintains or slightly increases the SVR, which will prevent right-to-left shunting. The disadvantage is that it may also slightly increase PVR, and in order to administer nitrous oxide, the FiO_2 needs to be reduced. A reduced FiO_2 may result in hypoxemia, which also results in an increase in PVR.

Blood Therapy

Question 8

Will you have blood in the room for this patient?

Answer 8

Yes. It is necessary to have blood in the room prior to incision. This is a major surgery with the potential for major bleeding.

C. Postoperative Care

Extubation

Question 1

Would you extubate this patient at the end of the case?

Answer 1

No. This patient has undergone a major cardiac operation and is also at risk for sudden death due to cardiac causes. Thus, I would want to reduce the work of breathing on this patient by maintaining her on a ventilator overnight and weaning her slowly in the following days.

Hypothermia

Question 2

Upon arrival to the PICU, the nurse tells you that the patient's temperature is 33°C. What will you do?

Answer 2

I would place a Bair hugger on the patient and administer warm fluids through a fluid warmer. I would also place some heated blankets around her head and have the PACU itself warmed.

Question 3

What are some harmful effects of hypothermia?

Answer 3

Hypothermia causes a number of deleterious effects, including hyperglycemia due to a decrease in plasma insulin, decreased intravascular volume due to cold-induced diuresis, decreased platelet function, and decreased drug metabolism.

Hypoxia

Question 4

On postoperative day #1 you notice during a routine postoperative visit that the patient's oxygen saturation is 85% on 40% FiO_2. The PICU intern said he turned down the FiO_2 because he was worried about retinopathy of prematurity (ROP). How do you respond?

Answer 4

I would inform the intern that ROP is only a consideration up to 44 weeks' postgestational age. This patient is already 6 months old and therefore outside of the window during which ROP can appear. I would further inform the intern that this patient needs to have adequate oxygenation because hypoxia will reduce oxygenation to this patient's tissues and may delay healing. The patient's FiO_2 should only be lowered if she is able to maintain adequate oxygen saturation at the lowered FiO_2.

Question 5

What will you do?

Answer 5

I will immediately place the patient on 100% O_2, check ETT position, and send an ABG to assess for other respiratory variables to ensure the patient is adequately ventilating and perfusing her tissues.

Suggested Readings

Hines RL, Marschall KE. *Stoelting's Anesthesia and Coexisting Disease.* Philadelphia: Churchill Livingstone; 2008.

Stoelting RK, Miller RD. *Basics of Anesthesia.* Philadelphia: Churchill Livingstone, 2007.

23 Neurological: Intracranial Mass

Sergey Pisklakov

Stem 1

A 65-year-old, 88 kg male is emergently scheduled for a posterior fossa intracranial tumor resection in the sitting position.

History of present illness: He has a 1-month history of increasing somnolence, headaches, aphasia, gait disturbances, and left-sided weakness.

Past medical history: The patient has history of chronic hypertension, cigarette smoking, and hypercholesterolemia.

Medications: He is taking HCTZ and Procardia.

Physical exam: Vital signs: BP 196/81 mmHg, pulse 74 bpm, RR 15, O_2 96% on RA.

Neurological: There is moderate bilateral papilledema. The rest of the exam is unremarkable.

Cardiovascular: RRR.

Lungs: CTA.

EKG: Normal sinus rhythm.

Studies: His head CT scan shows a posterior fossa lesion with mass effect.

Labs: Hb 11.8 g/dL.

A. Preoperative Evaluation

Neurological

Question 1

Does this patient have increased intracranial pressure (ICP)?

Answer 1

Yes. Gradually increasing somnolence, headache, papilledema, and mass effect on head CT are markers for increased ICP. The most important thing is to rule out Cushing's triad (bradypnea, bradycardia, and hypertension). Other markers for increased ICP are nausea, vomiting, headache, and ocular palsies.

Question 2

What is cerebral perfusion pressure?

Answer 2

Cerebral perfusion pressure is mean arterial pressure (MAP) – right atrial pressure (RAP) or ICP, whichever is greater.

Question 3

What premedication would you give to this patient in the holding area to alleviate anxiety?

Answer 3

Given the fact that this patient is experiencing increased somnolence, I would not suspect anxiety would be a major concern. I would refrain from giving any anxiolytic at this time. An anxiolytic such as a benzodiazepine carries the risk of compounding the somnolence and decreasing the respiration, which will increase the CO_2 levels and can lead to possible loss of the airway. Instead, I would reassess the patient, looking at the vital signs, and perform a focused neurological examination for any acute changes from baseline.

Cardiac

Question 4

How would you evaluate the patient's elevated blood pressure?

Answer 4

Assuming the patient is compliant with his antihypertensive medications, the elevated blood pressure is secondary to the elevated ICP. I would evaluate the elevated blood pressure by following the ICP trends, serial head CT for progression of the mass effect, and responses to mannitol and furosemide.

Question 5

How will you manage this patient's blood pressure preoperatively?

Answer 5

It is the elevated blood pressure that is permitting adequate cerebral perfusion in response to an elevated ICP. Thus, the first step in treating the blood pressure is actually lowering the ICP. I would make sure the patient's airway is not obstructed and that he is adequately oxygenating and ventilating. Next, I would elevate the patient's head 30 degrees, have the neurosurgeon drain some CSF, and administer mannitol or furosemide. If this was not successful, I would need to place the patient on mechanical ventilation and hyperventilate to decrease the $PaCO_2$.

Question 6

Do you need an echocardiogram in this patient?

Answer 6

Yes, if I hear a heart murmur on auscultation. Patients with intracardiac shunts such as ventral or atrial septal defect (VSD/ASD), ventriculoatrial shunts, or pulmonary arteriovenous malformations (AVMs) are contraindicated for the sitting position. Thus, I would want a baseline echocardiogram to rule out these cardiac lesions.

Position

Question 7

Surgery is to be performed in the sitting position. What are the benefits and drawbacks to a sitting position?

Answer 7

Benefits (reasons) for selecting the sitting position are as follows:

1. Better surgical exposure
2. Less tissue retraction and damage
3. Less bleeding
4. Less cranial nerve damage
5. More complete resection of the lesion
6. Early warning of venous air embolism and brainstem compromise
7. Less facial swelling
8. Ability to observe facial nerve function

Drawbacks (hazards) to patients being in the sitting position are as follows:

1. Venous air embolism
2. Hypotension
3. Vital sign changes secondary to brain stem manipulation
4. Cranial nerve stimulation (V, VII, X, XI)
5. Airway obstruction
6. Excessive neck flexion may cause quadriplegia from cervical spine ischemia.

Question 8

What are the main advantages of furosemide over mannitol at reducing the ICP?

Answer 8

Furosemide has several advantages over mannitol:

1. Furosemide does not increase cerebral blood volume (CBV) or ICP.
2. It can be used in CHF and/or renal patients.
3. It can be used in patients in whom the blood–brain barrier is compromised.

B. Intraoperative Management

Monitors

Question 1

What kind of monitoring is appropriate for this patient?

Answer 1

I would use the standard ASA monitors, a preinduction arterial line to monitor hemodynamics closely, a CVP for fluid assessment and for treatment of a venous air embolism (VAE), and possibly a TEE or precordial Doppler ultrasound for detection of a VAE.

Question 2

What monitors could you use to evaluate cerebral function?

Answer 2

Several monitors exist, none of which have been consistently shown to improve outcome: electroencephalography (EEG), processed EEG, somatosensory evoked potential (SSEP), transcranial Doppler ultrasound, and cerebral oximetry.

Question 3

How would you monitor this patient for venous air embolism?

Answer 3

It is suggested that precordial Doppler ultrasound in conjunction with expired CO_2 monitoring will fulfill this criteria for monitoring VAE. The transesophageal echo is slightly more sensitive in detecting clinical VAE events and is much more sensitive in detecting micro-bubbles in agitated saline. End-tidal nitrogen concentrations would only be able to detect a catastrophic VAE. In addition, the ventilator and breathing circuit would need to be absolutely free from air contamination. Transcranial Doppler ultrasound will detect air in the cerebral arteries. Its role is currently being evaluated. An esophageal stethoscope will detect a continuous or "mill-wheel" murmur with a severe VAE.

Positioning

Question 4

What are your concerns regarding a sitting position?

Answer 4

My concerns are the following:

1. Neck hyperflexion and cervical dislocation
2. External pressure on the eyes from the headrest

3. Poor visualization, access, and confirmation of the ETT and breathing circuit
4. Airway and/or jugular venous compression
5. Cerebral ischemia

Anesthesia Plan

Question 5

What are your main intraoperative considerations for this case?

Answer 5

The considerations are as follows:

1. The absolute avoidance of further increases in ICP
2. The provision of intraoperative brain relaxation to facilitate surgical access to the tumor
3. Maintaining stable hemodynamics to ensure adequate cerebral perfusion pressure

Question 6

What are your main goals during induction? How will you achieve it?

Answer 6

The main goals during induction of anesthesia are to avoid sudden increases in ICP, maintain adequate cerebral perfusion pressure, and avoid cerebral herniation.

I can achieve these goals by having the surgeon preemptively drain CSF through the external ventricular drain and administering mannitol or Lasix prior to induction. Assuming a normal airway, I would preoxygenate with 100% oxygen and perform a rapid sequence induction with lidocaine, fentanyl, etomidate, and rocuronium. I would pay close attention to the preinduction A-line and EKG for VS swings and be prepared to treat them with vasopressors and vasodilators.

Question 7

Can you use succinylcholine for induction?

Answer 7

Yes. However, I would be hesitant to administer succinylcholine because of possible further increases, albeit transient, in ICP. If the patient has a reassuring airway, a nondepolarizer such as rocuronium would be a better choice. If, however, this patient had a difficult airway, then the airway would take precedence over the ICP and I would use succinylcholine.

Question 8

What agents would you choose for maintenance in this patient? Why?

Answer 8

I would use a balanced technique with fentanyl, isoflurane, and rocuronium. Fentanyl and rocuronium offer the advantage of being cardiac stable, though copious amounts may lead to respiratory depression and delayed awakening. Isoflurane is easily titratable and may offer cerebral protection from the increased ICP.

Question 9

What are the effects of volatile anesthetics on ICP? What about IV anesthetics?

Answer 9

Volatile anesthetics increase cerebral blood flow (CBF) and may increase ICP. This effect is significantly exaggerated with persistent hypercarbia. CBF increases linearly with increases in $PaCO_2$ during isoflurane anesthesia and the combination of a volatile anesthetic and hypercarbia can result in higher levels of CBF than with either alone. Intravenous drugs, such as propofol, barbiturates, midazolam, and fentanyl, decrease CBF. They also result in a preservation of a linear CBF responsiveness to alterations in $PaCO_2$.

Maintenance

Question 10

What solution would be the best for intraoperative fluid management?

Answer 10

All infusions should be prepared with normal saline unless incompatible. Glucose-containing solutions promote cerebral edema and should not be used. Lactated Ringer's solutions, though widely used as the replacement fluid in neurosurgical patients, is hypotonic and therefore not as desirable.

Question 11

As the surgery begins, you notice changes to the somatosensory evoked potential? What will you do?

Answer 11

I would look at the monitors and make sure the patient is not hypoxic, hyper- or hypocarbic, or hypotensive and that the MAC value is less than 0.5. Next, I would rule out profuse bleeding, as anemia can also cause such changes. I would then inform the surgeon of these changes, after ruling out artifacts as the cause from the technician.

Question 12

The issue is now resolved. After 20 minutes, the surgeon complains of a "tight dura." How can you help?

Answer 12

Therapeutic maneuvers to Improve a "tight brain" are as follows:

1. Elevate head slightly to improve venous return
2. Hyperventilate
3. Check oxygenation
4. Check anesthetic agent; possibly need to turn off volatile agent
5. Give propofol to decrease CBV and decrease ICP
6. Give muscle relaxants to decrease ICP and improve venous return
7. Give diuretics to decrease brain edema
8. Spinal fluid drainage
9. Give additional steroids
10. Check for intracranial air. If present, pneumocephalus should be aspirated and nitrous oxide discontinued.

Question 13

Thirty minutes into the case, you notice a sudden drop in $EtCO_2$, hypotension, and tachycardia. What do you think is happening?

Answer 13

This sequelae points to a likely venous air embolism.

Question 14

What are you going to do about this?

Answer 14

I would:

1. Immediately inform the surgeon and call for help.
2. Promptly switch to 100% oxygen.
4. Have the surgeon irrigate the operative field with saline.
5. Have the surgeon occlude bone edges with wax to prevent further entrance of air.
6. Institute gentle compression of the jugular veins.
7. Aspirate air from the central venous catheter.
8. Provide hemodynamic support.

C. Postoperative Care

Hypertension

Question 1

The patient was brought to the PACU intubated. One hour later, you notice the BP is 190/100 mmHg. How will you respond?

Answer 1

I would immediately go to the bedside and confirm that this is an accurate reading while performing a focused neurological exam and assessing the other vital signs to rule out hypoxia, hypercarbia, or a malignant rhythm. Next, assuming these were normal, I would further assess for the cause, such as an elevated ICP, pain, or inadequate sedation. If all of these were normal and the hypertension was an isolated finding, I would infuse a vasodilator, such as nitroglycerin.

Peripheral Nerve Injury

Question 2

On the third postoperative day, you are told by your resident that the patient is complaining of difficulty dorsiflexing his left foot. How do you respond?

Answer 2

I would immediately go to the bedside and perform a focused history and physical. From the history, I would check the anesthesia record to make sure that the pressure points were adequately padded, specifically areas around the sciatic nerve. I would also ask the patient if he noticed this as soon as he awoke after the surgery or if this started later and whether there is concomitant pain or loss of sensation. From the physical, I would perform a focused neurological exam and assess for any other nerve palsies. I would also evaluate for any signs of inflammation, such as rubor, calor, or dolor.

Question 3

How would you treat this?

Answer 3

Assuming this was from a sciatic nerve injury, I would order electromyograms (EMGs) and nerve conduction studies and refer the patient for a neurological consultation. I would also reassure the patient that most of these cases resolve within 6–12 weeks and that he should follow up with a neurologist.

Suggested Readings

Cottrell JE, Young WL. *Cottrell's Neuroanesthesia*. 5th ed. St. Louis, MO: Elsevier Health Sciences; 2010.

Newfield P, Cottrell J. *Handbook of Neuroanesthesia*. 5th ed. Philadelphia: Lippincott Williams & Wilkins; 2012.

24 Neurological: Cerebral Aneurysm

Sergey Pisklakov

Stem 2

A 55-year-old 78 kg female is emergently scheduled for subarachnoid hemorrhage (SAH) evacuation and intracranial aneurysm clipping. She has a history of a previously diagnosed intracranial aneurysm and was already scheduled for elective intracranial aneurysm clipping. She also has a history headaches, coronary artery disease, hypertension, cigarette smoking, asthma, and hypercholesterolemia. She is awake and alert, but with a severe headache. Her BP is 176/80 mmHg, pulse 84 bpm, RR 15, O_2 96% on RA. She is currently on metoprolol, lipitor, and hydrochlorothiazide (HCTZ). She occasionally takes an albuterol inhaler for her asthma.

A. Preoperative Evaluation

Neurological

Question 1

How would you evaluate this patient's neurological status?

Answer 1

First, I would perform a history and physical. From the history, I would want to know this patient's baseline neurological status, including possible signs of increased intracranial pressure (ICP): somnolence, tiredness, mentation difficulties, worsening headache, nausea, and vomiting. From the physical, I would first assess her vital signs. Specifically, I would be concerned if there was hypertension with bradycardia and bradypnea, as this can be the Cushing's reflex, which is indicative of elevated ICP. I would also assess global and focal neurological deficits. Finally, I would look at any imaging studies that are available, such as a CT or MRI, which may help delineate the size of the hemorrhage.

Question 2

What are the normal values of cerebral blood flow (CBF)?

Answer 2

Total CBF in adults is about 50 mL/100 mg.

Question 3

What are the determinants of cerebral blood flow?

Answer 3

1. $PaCO_2$. Changes in $PaCO_2$ produce corresponding directional changes in CBF. CBF changes 1 mL/100 g/min for every 1 mmHg change in CO_2 from 40 mmHg. An increase of CO_2 from 40 to 80 mmHg doubles CBF, whereas a decrease to 20 halves it. Above and below those levels the CBF response plateaus
2. PaO_2. Decreases in PaO_2 do not produce significant increases in CBF until a threshold of 50 mmHg is present
3. pH, neuromediators, and neuromodulators
4. Neurogenic control
5. Temperature
6. Hematocrit

Question 4

What is meant by cerebral autoregulation? How does chronic hypertension affect this curve?

Answer 4

CBF remains constant between mean arterial pressures of 50 mmHg and 150 mmHg. This is termed cerebral autoregulation. Chronic hypertension shifts the autoregulatory curve to the right such that higher mean arterial pressures are tolerated before CBF becomes pressure dependent.

Question 5

The patient complains of a moderate headache and presents with nuchal rigidity. According to the Hunt and Hess classification, what grade is her hemorrhage?

Answer 5

According to the Hunt and Hess system, she would be a grade 2 hemorrhage.

Cardiac

Question 6

How does this patient's history of hypertension affect your anesthetic preparation?

Answer 6

Hypertension is a multisystem disease. It is important to know what organ systems are affected in this patient.

Neurological—hypertension shifts the cerebral autoregulatory curve to the right. I would avoid lowering the BP to more than 20% of baseline. I would also avoid lowering BP significantly, so as to not compromise cerebral perfusion pressure.

Cardiac—prolonged hypertension leads to left ventricular hypertrophy and increased myocardial work load. Conversely, even mild hypotension in this patient may have severe consequences because it may impair supply to already diseased myocardium.

Renal—hypertension can be a cause of renal failure, thus I would obtain a BUN/Cr to assess renal function.

Question 7

A preoperative EKG shows T-wave flattening with U waves. Are you concerned?

Answer 7

I would be less concerned if she does not complain of chest pains or demonstrate dysrhythmias since these EKG abnormalities appear preoperatively in 60% of patients who have SAH. The EKG alterations are most likely due to increased vagal and sympathetic neural output secondary to SAH. The changes are frequently T-wave inversions or flattening, ST segment depression or elevation, U waves, and QT interval prolongation.

Question 8

What will you do about the EKG findings?

Answer 8

I would want to compare the current EKG with a prior one. If these changes are new, I would need to distinguish the etiology as either SAH or cardiac. To rule out a cardiac etiology. I would look for signs and symptoms of a myocardial infarction, such as chest pains, shortness of breath, or diaphoresis.

Question 9

Would you delay the case?

Answer 9

No, because an active SAH is a true surgical emergency.

Question 10

What labs, if any, would you want before taking this patient to the OR?

Answer 10

I would want a baseline CBC, basic metabolic panel, and a type and cross for four units of PRBCs.

B. Intraoperative Management

Anesthesia

Question 1

What are your main hemodynamic goals during induction?

Answer 1

My goals during induction are to avoid abrupt changes in BP to ensure adequate coronary and cerebral perfusion while avoiding increasing the BP, which may further rupture the aneurysm.

Question 2

How will you achieve these goals?

Answer 2

To achieve these goals I would have in place a preinduction A-line and large-bore IVs and plan for a rapid sequence induction with cricoid pressure using etomidate, fentanyl, and succinycholine. Pressors and vasodilators would be placed on standby to help maintain the hemodynamic equilibrium.

Question 3

Immediately after induction, the BP suddenly plummets to 70/40 mmHg. What are you going to do?

Answer 3

I would check the patient's oxygenation and recycle the BP to make sure this was an accurate reading. I would next look at the EKG tracing to make sure this was not a malignant rhythm. Assuming all of these parameters were normal, I would open the fluids and give a low dose of a vasopressor such as phenylephrine to improve the BP.

Monitors

Question 4

What kind of monitoring are you going to use in this patient?

Answer 4

In addition to the standard ASA monitors (pulse oximetry, BP, EKG, $EtCO_2$, and temperature probe), a preinduction arterial line and Foley catheter are necessary.

Question 5

What monitors, if any, could you use to evaluate cerebral function? Which is the best?

Answer 5

There is no best monitor to evaluate for cerebral function. Several monitors exist, but none of these have been consistently shown to improve outcome: EEG, processed EEG, SSEP, transcranial Doppler, cerebral oximetry, jugular venous O_2 saturation, and stump pressures.

Question 6

What is the role of evoked potential monitoring in this case?

Answer 6

Evoked potentials are used to monitor the integrity of specific sensory and motor pathways. Sensory evoked potentials (SEPs) evaluate the functional integrity of ascending sensory pathways, whereas motor-evoked potentials (MEPs) test the functional integrity of descending motor pathways. All anesthetics that have been studied influence evoked potentials to some extent. Physiological factors such as temperature, BP, PaO_2, and $PaCO_2$ can substantially alter evoked potentials and must be controlled during intraoperative recording.

Question 7

You decide to use EEG monitoring. How does this affect your choice of drugs for maintenance?

Answer 7

In order to avoid interference with EEG monitoring, I have to make sure I use volatile agents in the value of 0.5 MAC or less.

Blood Pressure Control

Question 8

During manipulation of the aneurysm, the surgeon asks you to lower the BP. How do you respond? What is a major conflicting goal with the surgeon's request?

Answer 8

I would immediately look at the vital signs, paying close attention to the BP, HR, and EKG. Assuming the patient was otherwise stable, I would gently lower the BP up to 20% of baseline while paying close attention to any EKG changes. My conflicting goal here is lowering the BP to decrease the transmural pressure while maintaining the coronary perfusion pressure sufficient to prevent this patient from developing a myocardial infarction.

Question 9

Is there something you can ask the surgeon to do to decrease the transmural pressure across the aneurysm?

Answer 9

Yes. I can ask the surgeon to place a clip on the feeding vessel of the aneurysm.

Question 10

The surgeon places a temporary clip on the feeding vessel. How would this affect your management?

Answer 10

Now that the clip is in place, a higher than baseline BP must be maintained to support collateral blood flow to the cerebral tissues.

Question 11

Can you institute any other measures to offer cerebral protection?

Answer 11

Yes, I can administer barbiturates, which are protective in focal cerebral ischemia because they reduce $CMRO_2$ by reducing cerebral electrical activity. I can also institute hypothermia because doing so will decrease the rate of all metabolic reactions in cerebral tissue. Of course, decreasing the occlusion time and maintaining a higher baseline BP are very efficacious.

C. Postoperative Care

Rebleeding and Vasospasm

Question 1

What are your main concerns in the first 12 hours after the operation?

Answer 1

The most important considerations in SAH are rebleeding and vasospasm:

1. Rebleeding
   Recurrent hemorrhage from an aneurysm is the most devastating complication. It carries a high morbidity and mortality.
   Should rebleeding occur, the most important step is to control the ICP, with an immediate twist drill ventriculostomy and mannitol (1.0 g/kg IV). The risk of further hemorrhage is increased after a recurrent hemorrhage. A second bleed is often an indication for immediate surgery.
2. Vasospasm
   Reactive narrowing of the cerebral arterial tree after an SAH occurs in 30% of patients. Treatment for vasospasm includes the following:

   1) Hypervolemia (pulmonary capillary wedge pressure [PCWP] = 18 mmHg; central venous pressure [CVP] = 12 mmHg)
   2) Hemodilution (crit low in the 30s)
   3) Induced hypertension

Question 2

The surgeon asks you to extubate this patient on postoperative day #1. How do you respond?

Answer 2

My decision to extubate would depend on her intraoperative course. Assuming there has been no rebleeding, the original SAH was small and is evacuated, and cerebral edema is minimal, I would extubate. If, however, there is a high likelihood of cerebral edema and/or there was an intraoperative complication such as rebleeding, I would leave the patient sedated and intubated in the ICU and wait for the cerebral edema to decrease until I can comfortably extubate.

Question 3

During a routine postoperative visit, you notice the BP is 190/90 mmHg. How do you respond?

Answer 3

I would immediately go to the bedside and confirm that this is an accurate reading while assessing the other vital signs to rule out hypoxia, hypercarbia, or a malignant rhythm including myocardial infarction. Next, I would perform a focused neurological and pupillary exam. Assuming these were normal, I would further assess for the cause, such as anxiety. If no clear etiology could be determined, I may not need to treat because hypertension is used for treatment of vasospasm.

Postoperative Hyponatremia

Question 4

The next postoperative day, the patient's serum sodium reads 123 mEq/dL. What are the probable causes?

Answer 4

Possible causes include the syndrome of inappropriate antidiuretic hormone (SIADH) and cerebral salt wasting syndrome (CSWS). This occurs as a result of the release of atrial natriuretic peptide. CSWS is characterized by the triad of hyponatremia, volume contraction, and low to normal urine osmolarity. SIADH is characterized by hyponatremia in which the urine is hyperosmolar relative to the plasma. Clinically, SIADH patients are hypervolemic whereas CSWS patients are hypovolemic.

Suggested Readings

Cottrell JE, Young WL, eds. *Cottrell's Neuroanesthesia*. 5th ed. St. Louis, MO: Elsevier Health Sciences; 2010.

Newfield P, Cottrell J, eds. *Handbook of Neuroanesthesia*. 5th ed. Philadelphia, PA: Lippincott Williams & Wilkins; 2012.

25 Thoracic: VATS (One-Lung Ventilation)

Ruchir Gupta

Stem 1

A 71-year-old 64 kg, 5'7" female is scheduled for video-assisted thoracic surgery (VATS) to remove a right upper lobe carcinoma.

Past medical history: Asthma, COPD, HTN, hypercholesterolemia, CAD with stents.

Physical exam: BP 152/74 mmHg, pulse 63 bpm, RR 15, RA saturation 93%.

On physical exam, there is digital clubbing and moderate expiratory wheezing.

EKG: NSR, Q waves in II, III, aVF.

Echocardiogram: Left ventricular ejection fraction (LVEF) 48%.

Labs: Hct = 54%.

A. Preoperative Evaluation

Respiratory Function

Question 1

How would you evaluate this patient's respiratory status?

Answer 1

I would start with a focused history and physical. From the history, I would want to know this patient's baseline exercise tolerance, any shortness of breath at rest, compliance with home oxygen therapy, any prior anesthetics or intubations, and any problems weaning off the ventilator. I would also ask if there were any recent changes to her medicines for her COPD. From the physical, I would assess whether she is using any accessory muscle for breathing, any additional abnormalities on auscultation besides her wheezing, and whether she is tachypneic. Finally, I would evaluate any studies that may be available to me, such as an EKG to assess any right ventricular hypertrophy from her COPD, a baseline chest X-ray, and any PFTs.

Question 2

Does this patient need PFTs?

Answer 2

I would not require PFTs in this patient. A focused history and physical can provide me with the information that I need: disease severity, possible dependence on home oxygen, response to bronchodilators, exacerbating or alleviating factors, and baseline exercise tolerance.

Question 3

What would you expect her ABG to show?

Answer 3

I would expect a compensated respiratory acidosis with hypoxia. The plasma bicarbonate level would likely be elevated as a compensatory mechanism against the elevated $PaCO_2$.

Cyanosis

Question 4

What do you think of the patient's Hct level and digital clubbing? Are they related?

Answer 4

Yes, they are related because both can occur with chronic hypoxia. Chronic hypoxia can lead to erythrocytosis and pulmonary HTN with subsequent right heart failure. Though the mechanism is unclear, cyanosis can lead to an overgrowth of connective tissue and result in digital clubbing.

B. Intraoperative Management

Monitoring

Question 1

How would you monitor this patient?

Answer 1

I would use the standard ASA monitors with a 5-lead EKG as well as a preinduction A-line to monitor closely the hemodynamic changes during induction. I would also want a Foley catheter.

Epidural Catheter Placement

Question 2

Assuming this patient stopped clopidogrel 4 days ago, would you place a thoracic epidural for postoperative pain control?

Answer 2

No. Placement of an epidural catheter is contraindicated because of the risk of bleeding. The American Society of Regional Anesthesiology (ASRA) guidelines require clopidogrel to be held for 7 days before performing an epidural, assuming normal renal and hepatic function. In addition, the case will need to be delayed for an additional 3 days for normal platelet function to resume.

Question 3

How does clopidogrel work?

Answer 3

Clopidogrel is an adenosine 5′-diphosphate (ADP) receptor inhibitor. ADP receptors play an important role in the activation of platelets.

Question 4

Assuming that she was on aspirin (ASA) instead of clopidogrel, would you place an epidural catheter?

Answer 4

Yes. According to the ASRA guidelines, ASA does not increase the risk of a neuraxial hematoma.

Induction

Question 5

How would you induce this patient?

Answer 5

Assuming she has a reassuring airway, I would perform a slow, controlled induction using fentanyl, lidocaine, etomidate, and, once the ability to ventilate has been established, rocuronium.

Endotracheal Tube

Question 6

What type of endotracheal tube (ETT) will you use?

Answer 6

A left-sided double-lumen tube (DLT) is preferable as it provides a greater margin for error in positioning. Ventilation of the right upper lobe can be a challenge with a right-sided DLT because of its proximity to the carina.

Question 7

What are the absolute and relative indications for DLTs?

Answer 7

The absolute indications or DLTs are bronchopulmonary lavage, bronchopleurocutaneous fistula, lung abscess, bronchial hemorrhage, giant air cyst, or a communicating empyema.

Relative indications are divided into high-priority surgical exposure (pneumonectomy, upper lobectomy, thorocoabdominal aneurysm repair) and low-priority surgical exposure (esophageal resection, middle and lower lobectomy).

Question 8

Your bronchoscope isn't functioning well so you decide to use the "clamp" technique to verify the location of your DLT. Upon inflation of both cuffs and clamping of the tracheal lumen, you hear bilateral breath sounds. What are you going to do?

Answer 8

Presence of bilateral breath sounds after clamping of the tracheal lumen implies that bilateral ventilation is occurring through the bronchial lumen. This can only be possible if the bronchial lumen is in the trachea and not the left bronchus as desired. Thus, I would attempt to push my DLT in further, directing my bronchial lumen into the left main bronchus.

Ventilation

Question 9

The patient was placed in the lateral decubitus position. What effect does this position have on ventilation?

Answer 9

The lateral decubitus position results in greater V/Q mismatch because blood is preferentially directed to the dependent lung while oxygenation is preferentially directed to the nondependent lung.

Hypoxia

Question 10

Twenty minutes into one-lung ventilation (OLV), the patient's oxygen saturation decreases to 93% despite being on 100% oxygen. How do you respond?

Answer 10

I would immediately check the other vital signs to make sure the patient is not hypercarbic, hypotensive, or in a malignant arrhythmia, and 100% oxygen would be maintained. Proper DLT positioning would be confirmed by auscultating the chest while manually providing bag ventilation. Direct visualization with fiber-optic bronchoscopy would also be used. If that didn't work, I would apply CPAP to the nondependent lung and then if still unsuccessful, add PEEP to the ventilated lung. Finally, if all of these measures failed, I would reinflate the nondependent lung and discuss temporary pulmonary artery clamping with the surgeon.

Question 11

What if the saturation had dropped to 85% despite your measures?

Answer 11

This is a more catastrophic drop in saturation, and I would not want to delay restoring the saturation using the aforementioned techniques. Thus, while checking the other vital signs, I would notify the surgeon that I am immediately restoring two lung ventilation.

Massive Bleeding

Question12

Hypoxemia issues resolve. Thirty minutes later, you notice that the patient suddenly develops hypotension with a BP of 72/47 mmHg. What will you do?

Answer 12

I would recheck the BP immediately by looking at my arterial-line tracing and recycling the noninvasive BP cuff. I would also check the other vital signs, making sure the patient is not hypoxic, hypocarbic, or in a malignant arrhythmia. Assuming these were normal, I would open the fluids wide open and communicate with the surgical team, examining the surgical field for active bleeding or other acute event. I would immediately call for blood and administer low doses of a pressor as a temporizing measure.

C. Postoperative Care

Extubation

Question 1

With bleeding under control at the end of the case, would you extubate this patient if the vital signs are stable?

Answer 1

No. Given the volume of intraoperative blood transfusion, fluid shifts, and her preoperative COPD status, I would opt to leave this patient intubated in the ICU while her fluid status improves.

Question 2

You decide to leave this patient intubated. Your resident asks if you should switch to a single-lumen tube (SLT). How do you respond?

Answer 2

I would tell the resident that I will switch to a SLT because it is less bulky and therefore more comfortable for the patient, causes less edema and necrosis, and usually is easier to manage by ICU nurses who may not have experience with DLTs. In addition, DLTs have a propensity to reposition more readily than SLTs.

Question 3

The patient is now in the ICU and an ABG drawn by your resident shows the following: pH 7.30 mmHg, PaO_2 70 mmHg, $PaCO_2$ 55 mmHg, on 40% FiO_2. Please interpret these results.

Answer 3

This is respiratory acidosis with hypoxemia.

Question 4

What PaO_2 would you want on this patient with this FiO_2?

Answer 4

The ideal PaO_2 on 40% FiO_2 would be 200 mmHg (FiO_2 x 5).

Question 5

What will you do about this blood gas finding?

Answer 5

I would go immediately to the bedside, place the patient on 100% oxygen, and examine the patient. Specifically, I would evaluate whether this was due to issues with the ETT or with the patient's ventilation. I would check the position of the ETT, auscultate for bilateral breath sounds, and suction the ETT for any mucus plugs. Assuming all of these were normal, I would look at the patient's ventilation settings. If she was on synchronized intermittent mechanical ventilation (SIMV), I would conclude that she is unable to pull adequate tidal volumes on this setting, so I would change her to continuous mandatory ventilation (CMV) mode with PEEP and increase her tidal volume as needed. If she was already on CMV, I would look at her ventilation settings and consider increasing her tidal volume and/or respiratory rate.

Postoperative Pain Control

Question 6

What are some options for postoperative pain control in this patient?

Answer 6

There are several options for pain control in this patient. Assuming the patient is awake and extubated, a PCA would be helpful. The patient also can have regional nerve blocks such as intercostal nerve blocks, paravertebral nerve blocks, cryoneurolysis, and neuraxial techniques. Neuraxial techniques should be used with caution if this patient is on any anticoagulation for her cardiac stents.

Altered Mental Status

Question 7

The patient is successfully extubated on postoperative day #1. The ICU nurse pages you because the patient is confused and tachycardic. What is your approach?

Answer 7

I would go immediately to the bedside and make sure she is not hypoxic, hypercarbic, hypotensive, or in a malignant arrhythmia. I would then perform a focused history and physical. From the history, I would review the medications that the patient has received in the perioperative period, the medical chart for previously mentioned diagnoses, and the ICU notes to see what medications she has been given—specifically pain medicines, because they can cause delirium. The physical examination would include a focused neurological exam, including evaluation of her pupils. Finally, I would order stat labs including ABG, electrolytes, and glucose. If a stroke seemed possible, a stat head CT and neurology consult would be obtained.

Suggested Readings

Barash PG, Cullen BF, Stoelting RK, Cahalan M, Stock CM, eds. *Clinical Anesthesia.* 6th ed. Philadelphia, PA: Lippincott Williams & Wilkins; 2009.

Miller RD, Eriksson LI, Fleisher LA, Wiener-Kornish JP, Young WL, eds. *Miller's Anesthesia.* 7th ed. Philadelphia, PA: Churchill Livingstone Elsevier; 2010.

Yao F, Fontes ML, Malhotra V, eds. *Yao and Artusio's Anesthesiology: Problem-Oriented Patient Management.* 7th ed. Philadelphia, PA: Lippincott Williams & Wilkins; 2011.

26 Thoracic: Mediastinal Mass

Stanley Yuan and Joseph Marino

A 32-year-old male presents for biopsy of a mediastinal mass. He complains of difficulty swallowing for the past several weeks. His past medical history is significant for severe asthma. His medications include albuterol, pyridostigmine, and advair. Vital signs are HR 76 bpm, BP 112/67 mmHg, RR 14, O_2 saturation 96% RA. Hb = 11.4 g/dL, platelets = 290 K.

A. Preoperative Evaluation

Airway

Question 1

How would you evaluate the extent of this patient's mediastinal mass?

Answer 1

I would perform a full history and physical. I would want to know how long this patient has had dysphagia, progression of the symptoms, and aggravating or alleviating factors. I would also inquire about any signs of superior vena cava (SVC) syndrome such as headache, confusion, or altered mental status. From the physical exam I would look for any gross deviations in the oropharynx and for palpable masses in the neck. I would also look for signs of SVC syndrome such as facial cyanosis, venous distension of the neck or arm, and any edema of the upper extremity. Finally, imaging studies such as a CT or an MRI are valuable to determine the location and size of the mass as well as the degree of tracheal deviation.

Question 2

How does the presence of a mediastinal mass affect your anesthetic plan?

Answer 2

A mediastinal mass can result in airway and cardiovascular collapse. Depending on size and location, most of these cases are not amenable to local anesthesia. The primary goal of general anesthesia is to secure the airway while keeping the patient spontaneously breathing.

Question 3

Are flow-volume loops essential as part of the preoperative assessment? What about an echocardiogram?

Answer 3

No. Flow-volume loops have been shown to correlate poorly to the degree of airway obstruction and have not been useful in managing these types of patients. The most useful information comes from a history and physical exam as well as pertinent imaging studies. An echocardiogram would be indicated if there were additional symptoms such as shortness of breath or congestive heart failure. In the absence of these symptoms, I would not rush to order an echocardiogram at this time as it would not affect my management.

Asthma

Question 4

How would you assess this patient's asthma?

Answer 4

I would assess this patient's asthma by first performing a focused history and physical exam. From the history, I would elicit how long the patient has had asthma, whether he has ever had to go to the ER for an exacerbation, and whether he has had any hospitalizations or intubations as a result of the asthma. I would also want to know the aggravating and alleviating factors, degree of improvement from the inhaler, and any complications with past anesthetics. I would inquire about any recent chest colds or upper respiratory infections (URIs). From the physical exam I would assess to see if this patient is breathing comfortably, whether any accessory muscle use is occurring, and whether any wheezes or rhonchi are present. Finally, I would review any imaging studies, such as a chest X-ray, if they were available.

Endocrine Status

Question 5

Why is this patient on pyridostigmine?

Answer 5

As an anticholinesterase inhibitor, pyridostigmine is normally given to patients with myasthenia gravis since it is an autoimmune disease in which circulating antibodies bind to acetylcholine receptors, rendering them inactive. Pyridostigmine increases the concentration of circulating acetylcholine molecules, thereby increasing the probability at which acetylcholine binds to the receptors.

Question 6

How does pyridostigmine affect your anesthetic planning for this case?

Answer 6

The patient's chronic use of pyridostigmine may interfere with the ability to reverse this patient's paralysis. Thus, the patient may remain paralyzed for a prolonged period of time, necessitating the use of postoperative ventilation.

Question 7

Would you continue the pyridostigmine on the day of surgery?

Answer 7

Yes. I would tell the patient to continue his medication on the day of surgery and also inform him of the potential necessity of postoperative ventilator support.

B. Intraoperative Management

Induction

Question 1

What intraoperative monitors would you use for induction?

Answer 1

In addition to the standard ASA monitors, I would place an arterial line in the right radial artery to evaluate innominate artery compression during mediastinoscopy. I would want to have one pulse oximeter in the right upper extremity to diagnose right innominate artery compression and one in the lower extremity in case I lost my pulse oximeter tracing in the upper extremity during the procedure. For a large mediastinal mass, I would also consider placing bilateral femoral lines so that if life-threatening airway collapse occurred, cardiopulmonary bypass could be initiated.

Question 2

How would you induce this patient?

Answer 2

A discussion with the surgeon is needed to confirm that a rigid bronchoscope is immediately available and a sternal saw if life-threatening airway compromise occurs. I would preserve spontaneous ventilation and perform an awake fiber-optic intubation by topicalizing the airway using viscous lidocaine spray. If needed, I would titrate ketamine for its bronchodilatory effect and ability to maintain spontaneous ventilation.

Question 3

The patient refuses an awake fiber-optic intubation. Now what?

Answer 3

I would have a detailed discussion with the patient about the risks involved with his airway due to the mediastinal mass. I would continue to reassure him that this is the safest way. If he still doesn't allow me to perform an awake fiber-optic procedure, I would place all of my difficult-airway equipment on standby and perform an inhalational induction with sevoflurane while maintaining spontaneous ventilation.

Question 4

After securing the endotracheal tube (ETT), you suddenly lose the $EtCO_2$ tracing. How do you respond?

Answer 4

I would immediately manually ventilate the patient to assess compliance of the airway as well as provide positive pressure breaths with 100% oxygen. If I still couldn't ventilate or I suspected mass compression as the etiology, I would attempt to pass a rigid bronchoscope beyond the obstruction and move the patient in the lateral or prone position to relieve the compression on the airway. Finally, if none of these maneuvers were successful, I would ask the surgeon to open the chest and begin cardiopulmonary bypass.

Hypotension

Question 5

Your $EtCO_2$ returns and you are able to ventilate. The procedure begins uneventfully but 15 minutes into the case, the right arterial tracing is diminished during mediastinoscopy. What do you do?

Answer 5

This is usually due to compression of the innominate artery causing artificially low BP readings. I would check a radial or femoral pulse to rule out significant hypotension. I would also pay attention to the capnogram to rule out ventilation issues and the EKG to identify any dysrhythmias that may have occurred. Assuming that the flattening of the arterial tracing is due to the innominate artery compression, I would ask the surgeon to remove the mediastinoscope while palpating for a pulse in the left arm. If those measures failed, I would begin resuscitation with fluids, blood, and pressors to restore hemodynamics.

Question 6

What is the relevance of facial and upper extremity edema during mediastinoscopy?

Answer 6

Compression of the great vessels by a tumor in the anterior mediastinum can lead to SVC syndrome. This may reduce preload with severely decreased CO. Therefore, I would ensure adequate preload prior to induction, large-bore

IV access in the lower extremities, and arterial line placement in the right radial artery to diagnose innominate artery compression. Because of the compromised cardiac output, avoidance of positive pressure ventilation is also warranted.

Hypoxia

Question 7

Thirty minutes into the procedure, you lose your pulse oximeter reading. How do you respond? What is your differential?

Answer 7

I would immediately look at the other vital signs and make sure the patient is not hypotensive or hypocarbic and has not developed any arrhythmias. I would also listen for bilateral breath sounds to rule out pneumothorax, which is a recognized complication of mediastinoscopy. I would also take the patient off the ventilator and manually ventilate the patient to assess lung compliance. Concomitant loss of $ETCO_2$ would argue strongly for an airway obstruction, most likely due to mass compression on the airway. If that did not work, I would push my ETT and/or the rigid bronchoscope distal to the lesion in an attempt to relieve the compression. I would also lighten the anesthesia and awaken the patient. Ultimately, the patient may have to be turned laterally or prone to relieve the airway mass compression. If the arterial pressure also disappeared, this would most likely be innominate artery compression.

C. Postoperative Management

Extubation

Question 1

The surgeon wants a deep extubation in an effort to evaluate vocal cord function.
How do you respond?

Answer 1

My preference is to extubate the patient fully awake and assess vocal cord function postoperatively. My primary concern is to avoid loss of the airway.

Question 2

After neuromuscular block reversal, the patient manifests weakness and respiratory distress following extubation. What are the possible causes?

Answer 2

The patient could be experiencing hypoxia, hypercarbia, hypotension, or malignant arrhythmia. In addition, assuming this patient has myasthenia gravis as evidenced by the chronic pyridostigmine use, I would have to rule out a myasthenic versus cholinergic crisis. Administration of edrophonium would improve the weakness, affirming a myasthenic crisis; exacerbation of the weakness would confirm a cholinergic crisis and reintubation may be indicated. Other causes may be inadequate reversal of neuromuscular blocker, residual anesthetics, pneumothorax, pulmonary embolism, atelectasis, and pulmonary edema.

PACU

Question 3

The patient develops postoperative hoarseness in the PACU. How would you evaluate this?

Answer 3

I would go immediately to the bedside and rule out hypoxia, hypotension, hypocarbia, or malignant arrhythmia. My most immediate concern would be recurrent laryngeal nerve injury (a recognized complication of mediastinoscopy), laryngeal edema, tracheomalacia, residual neuromuscular paralysis, or myasthenic weakness. I would check twitches to assess muscle strength, go over my anesthetic record to see what doses of narcotics and anesthetics were given, and assess whether they have worn off. Nerve injury would be a diagnosis of exclusion. Depending on the vital signs and clinical picture, I would provide supplemental oxygen and have intubating equipment on standby.

Question 4

The patient developed a left-sided hemiparesis following the procedure. The surgeon asks if this could be a myasthenic crisis. How do you respond?

Answer 4

I would inform the surgeon that this is most likely not a myasthenic crisis because postoperative weakness from myasthenia gravis usually is global in nature. This focal deficit strongly points to a right-sided cerebrovascular event, most likely caused by intraoperative hypotension, air or hemorrhagic embolism, or cerebral ischemia from right innominate artery compression.

Suggested Readings

Gothard JWW. Anesthetic considerations for patients with anterior mediastinal masses. *Anesthesiol Clin.* 2008;26: 305–314

Slinger P, Karsil C. Management of patients with a large anterior mediastinal mass: recurring myths. *Curr Opin Anesthesiol.* 2007;20:1–3

27 Cardiovascular: Aortic Dissection

Ruchir Gupta

Stem 1

A 55-year-old male is brought to the OR for emergent repair of a thoracic aortic dissection.

History of present illness: The patient is an actor who, during rehearsal, complained of a nonspecific ripping chest pain that radiated to the neck.

Past medical history: Hypertension, hypercholesterolemia.

Medications: Enalapril, Lipitor.

Allergies: NKDA.

Physical exam: Vital signs: BP = 175/85 mmHg, HR = 120 bpm, RR = 18, O_2 saturation = 98% on 2 L/min O_2, T = 37°C.

Airway: Mallampati 3, thyromental distance <6 cm.

Cardiovascular: Tachycardic, 2/6 diastolic murmur.

Chest X-ray: Widened mediastinum.

Labs: Hct = 31%, coagulation profile is normal.

A. Preoperative Evaluation

Heart Murmur

Question 1

What do you think is the cause of the diastolic murmur in this patient?

Answer 1

Based on the information given, it is difficult to conclude definitively the cause of the murmur. If this is a new-onset murmur, then quite possibly the aortic dissection may be extending into the aortic valve and causing aortic regurgitation. However, if this diastolic murmur was present even before this event, then it can be from mitral or tricuspid stenosis.

Classification for Dissection

Question 2

Describe the Debakey classification system for aortic dissection.

Answer 2

The Debakey classification is as follows:

Type I begins in the ascending aorta and extending to the abdominal aorta.

Type II begins and remains in the ascending aorta.

Type III originates beyond the left subclavian artery and extends to the diaphragm (IIIA) or the aortoiliac bifurcation (IIIB).

Types I and II are considered surgical emergencies, whereas type III is a medical emergency.

Preoperative Assessment

Question 3

What further information regarding this patient's preoperative history would you want to know?

Answer 3

I would want to know more about this patient's cardiac, pulmonary, and renal status. For the cardiac assessment I would want to know whether this patient has had any recent stress tests or echocardiograms, any recent episodes of chest pain or dyspnea at rest, and whether his murmur is new or chronic. For the pulmonary history I would want to know if this patient is a smoker or has had any signs or symptoms of COPD, because this patient will most likely remain intubated postoperatively. Finally, the presence of renal dysfunction is the single most important predictor of the development of renal failure after surgery. Thus I would want a baseline BUN/creatinine test for this patient.

Question 4

If time permitted, would you want PFTs done in this patient?

Answer 4

No. The patient's respiratory status can be assessed with a thorough history and physical and I do not believe PFTs would give me any additional information that would affect my acute management.

OR Setup

Question 5

What instructions would you give your first-year anesthesia resident regarding OR setup for this case?

Answer 5

This is a case with a potential for massive blood loss and hemodynamic fluctuations. Thus, I would tell my resident to have the following items set up in the room: at least four NS-spiked IVs, four units of PRBCs typed and crossed in the room, with another four units on hold from the blood bank, a central line, TEE, an arterial line, a rapid transfuser, a cell saver, and a crash cart in the event defibrillation or cardioversion becomes necessary. I would also ask the resident to have nitroglycerin and norepinephrine drips set up in anticipation of the aortic cross-clamp.

B. Intraoperative Management

Monitoring

Question 1

How would you monitor this patient?

Answer 1

In addition to the standard ASA monitors, I would place a central line for volume resuscitation and CVP monitoring, a TEE to assess cardiac function, an arterial line for continuous BP monitoring as well as frequent ABGs, and a Foley catheter.

Question 2

Assuming you decide to place an arterial line, where would you place it?

Answer 2

I would not place one, but two arterial lines, so that I can assess the BP proximal and distal to the clamp. The proximal A-line would be placed in the right radial artery because the left subclavian artery may be clamped during the surgery, impairing blood flow to the left arm. The distal A-line could be placed in either femoral artery.

Airway

Question 3

How will you secure this patient's airway?

Answer 3

Since the patient likely has a difficult airway, I would perform an awake fiber-optic intubation (AFOI) with airway nerve blocks and adequate airway topicalization with 4% nebulized lidocaine. I would have a nitroglycerin drip on standby to prevent sudden blood pressure swings during the procedure.

Question 4

You decide to perform an AFOI, but as you are about to begin, the surgeon yells that there is no time for an AFOI. How would you respond?

Answer 4

I would inform the surgeon that there is no faster technique for securing the airway and that is also safe for a patient with a suspected difficult airway. Failure to secure the airway can result in apnea, hypoxia, and death. Thus, although this may be an emergency, it is important to do what is safe for the patient.

Question 5

You successfully intubate the patient. Thirty minutes later, the surgeon informs you that he will be placing the cross-clamp on the aorta in the next few minutes. What hemodynamic fluctuations should you prepare for?

Answer 5

The hemodynamic changes I would expect are as follows:

Proximal to the clamp: Increased afterload, increased BP to upper half of body, increased CVP and pulmonary artery occlusion pressure, and decreased CO and ejection fraction (EF)

Distal to the clamp: Decreased renal blood flow and mesenteric blood flow

Overall, there would be increased mixed venous oxygenation, decreased O_2 consumption, metabolic acidosis, and increased catecholamine release.

Aortic Cross-Clamp

Question 6

As soon as the surgeon places the cross-clamp, the BP rises to 210/110 mmHg. What are you going to do?

Answer 6

The desire to treat the abrupt increase in BP, which is most likely due to an acute increase in afterload, must be weighed against the risk of reducing perfusion pressure distal to the cross-clamp. Thus I would attempt to gently reduce the afterload with an infusion of nitrogylcerin or sodium nitroprusside while paying close attention to the perfusion pressure distal to the cross-clamp.

Question 7

Your resident begins a nitroglycerin infusion but the patient begins to develop tachycardia. What will you do?

Answer 7

I will have my resident stop the infusion because tachycardia is a known side effect of nitroglycerin. Instead, I will switch to an esmolol drip to lower the BP and the HR.

Question 8

As you lower the BP, your arterial line in the lower extremity gives you a reading of 75/45 mmHg while the proximal arterial line reading is still elevated. What will you do?

Answer 8

After confirming that both readings were accurate I would attempt to improve the perfusion pressure distal to the cross-clamp by asking the surgeon to place a shunt, reimplant arteries to perfuse vital organs such as the kidney, spinal cord, and liver, and institute hypothermia.

My target would be to try to maintain an MAP of 100 mmHg proximal to the clamp and 50 mmHg distal to the clamp.

Question 9

You are able to maintain stable hemodynamics during the cross-clamp portion of the surgery. The surgeon immediately removes the cross-clamp without telling you and the BP plummets to 70/40 mmHg. ST changes are noted on the EKG. What are you going to do?

Answer 9

I would instruct the surgeon to immediately reapply the clamp. Once the BP improves, I would ask him to slowly and incrementally remove the clamp while I begin an infusion of norepinephrine or phenylephrine to increase the patient's SVR and to tolerate the effects of unclamping.

C. Postoperative Care

Extubation

Question 1

Would you extubate this patient right after surgery?

Answer 1

I would not extubate this patient because he has undergone a major vascular operation with likely blood loss and massive fluid shifts. Additionally, the incision wound is quite painful and may impair his ventilation. Thus, the risks of extubation outweigh the benefits in this case. I would leave the patient intubated overnight and gradually wean him once his fluid shifts have stabilized.

Hypothermia

Question 2

Upon arrival in the PACU, the temperature is only 35°C. What are the immediate effects of hypothermia?

Answer 2

Hypothermia causes a number of deleterious effects, including hyperglycemia due to a decrease in plasma insulin, decreased volume due to cold-induced diuresis, decreased platelet functions, and decreased drug metabolism.

Question 3

How would you treat this patient's hypothermia?

Answer 3

I would place a Bair hugger on the patient and administer fluids through a fluid warmer. I would also place some heated blankets around his head and consider calling to have the PACU itself warmed.

Delayed Awakening

Question 4

You turn off all sedatives in an effort to awaken the patient over the course of the next several hours. However, the patient remains unresponsive. What will you do?

Answer 4

Delayed awakening in this patient can be a very ominous sign because the hemodynamic fluctuations could have resulted in ischemia to the brain and spinal cord. I would initially evaluate the patient to ensure he is not hypoxic, hypotensive, or in a malignant rhythm. After that, I would review the anesthesia chart as well as the nurse's notes to see what medicines were given, including pain medicine, that can still be lingering. I would check twitches to make sure the patient is adequately reversed. I would also send off labs including an ABG and electrolytes to make sure the patient is not hypoglycemic or anemic. Finally, if all of this was negative, I would send the patient for an emergent CT scan of the head.

Suggested Readings

Ghansah JN, Murphy JT. Complications of major aortic and lower extremity vascular surgery. *Semin Cardiothorac Vasc Anesth.* 2004;8(4):335–361.

Shine TS, Murray MJ. Intraoperative management of aortic aneurysm surgery. *Anesthesiol Clin North Am.* 2004;22(2):289–305.

Yao F, Fontes ML, Malhotra V, eds. *Yao and Artusio's Anesthesiology, Problem-Oriented Patient Management.* 7th ed. Philadelphia, PA: Lippincott Williams & Wilkins; 2011.

28 Cardiovascular: Carotid Endarterectomy

Ruchir Gupta

A 66-year old, 70 kg male is scheduled for a left carotid endarterectomy. He has a history of coronary artery disease, hypertension, and hypercholesterolemia. His BP is 126/80 mmHg, pulse 74 bpm, RR 15, SpO_2 96% on RA. He is currently on metoprolol, lipitor, and hydrochlorothiazide (HCTZ).

A. Preoperative Evaluation

Cardiac

Question 1

How would you evaluate this patient's cardiac status?

Answer 1

First, I would perform a history and physical. From the history, I would want to know what this patient's baseline exercise tolerance is as evidenced by how many flights of stairs he can climb before becoming short of breath. I would also ask him if he has any chest pain at rest. From the physical, I would want to know if there is evidence of fluid overload, such as JVD or pedal edema, which would strongly suggest congestive heart failure. I would also look at a recent EKG and compare it to an old one if available, and also look for the results of any echocardiogram and stress tests he may have had. I would also speak with his cardiologist if he or she were available.

Hypertension

Question 2

How does this patient's history of hypertension affect your anesthetic management?

Answer 2

Hypertension is a multisystem disease; therefore, it is important to know what organ systems are affected in this patient and then adjust the anesthetic plan accordingly.

Neurological: Hypertension shifts the cerebral autoregulatory curve to the right, so what would normally be acceptable at the lower range of MAP may not be applicable in this patient. Thus, I would avoid lowering the BP to more than 20% of baseline.

Cardiac: Prolonged untreated hypertension can lead to left ventricular hypertrophy (LVH) and increased myocardial work load. I would review the EKG to see if there was evidence of LVH.

Renal: Hypertension can be a cause of renal failure; thus, if there was evidence of renal compromise, I would avoid drugs that are renally excreted and check a K+ level.

Question 3

What if the patient came to the OR with a BP of 160/90 mmHg?

Answer 3

I would compare it to the patient's baseline, and if the BP is acutely elevated I would probe for the cause. If it is chronic, I would hesitate to lower it because if this patient has critical carotid stenosis, an elevated BP may be necessary to maintain cerebral perfusion. If it is acute, I would determine what the cause was; if anxiety, I would give midazolam; if pain, I would consider a pain reliever. I would also obtain a 12-lead EKG to rule out any myocardial events.

Question 4

What if the BP is 210/110 mmHg?

Answer 4

I would obviously be more concerned, as this is hypertensive emergency, defined as a diastolic blood pressure ≥120 mmHg and/or systolic blood pressure ≥180 mmHg. Although I would apply the same principles as mentioned in my previous response, I would be more aggressive in lowering this patient's BP with labetalol or even nitroglycerin.

Question 5

Are you concerned that lowering the BP from 210/100 mmHg may compromise cerebral perfusion?

Answer 5

It is unlikely that such an elevated BP is absolutely necessary to maintain cerebral perfusion. Although I would discuss with the surgeon the extent of this patient's carotid stenosis, I would certainly want to lower the BP somewhat because at this level the patient runs the risk of a hemorrhagic stroke. Additionally, given this patient's history of coronary artery disease, the increased afterload on the heart as a result of this BP will increase the workload on the heart and increase this patient's risk of a myocardial infarction.

Neurological

Question 6

Would you perform a neurological evaluation of this patient?

Answer 6

Yes, I would. Because this patient has a history of carotid stenosis, I would be interested to know if this patient has had any transient ischemic attacks (TIAs) or symptoms of stroke. If so, I would want to know if there is any muscle weakness or any other neurological sequelae from these incidents.

Question 7

Let's suppose the patient has right arm weakness from a stroke he suffered 2 years ago. How would that affect your anesthetic care?

Answer 7

If this patient had a stroke with a right arm weakness, I would avoid using that extremity for monitors such as a BP cuff or a twitch monitor and placement of IV lines. In addition, I would avoid giving this patient succinycholine, because I am worried about denervation sensitivity from the stroke causing life-threatening hyperkalemia in this patient.

B. Intraoperative Management

Anesthesia

Question 1

Would you use regional or general anesthetic for this case?

Answer 1

There is no clear preferred method here. The main benefit of regional anesthesia is that it provides us with an awake patient, which allows us to better monitor the cerebral and cardiac status of the patient. Additionally, hemodynamic instability associated with induction and maintenance of general anesthesia is avoided. The disadvantages of regional is the potential need for emergency intubation during the case, complications related to the cervical block, and possible patient movement during the case. The patient's anxiety level must also be assessed before administering regional anesthesia because extremely anxious patients may not be able to remain still for the duration of the case.

Question 2

If you did decided to do a regional procedure, which block would you use?

Answer 2

I would use a superficial and deep cervical block.

Question 3

What will you tell the patient are the possible complications related to the block?

Answer 3

I would tell the patient that there is a risk of nerve injury, a risk of bleeding by accidental puncture of a blood vessel, a risk of intravascular injection, a risk that the needle might enter the epidural space and cause a high regional, and a risk that other nerves could be blocked, causing a Horner's syndrome or hemiparalysis of the diaphragm. All of these would be in addition to the risk of the nerves not being properly blocked, making a general anesthetic necessary.

Monitors

Question 4

What kind of monitoring are you going to use in this patient?

Answer 4

In addition to the standard ASA monitors (pulse oximeter, noninvasive BP, EKG, $EtCO_2$, and temperature), I would want to have an arterial line to closely and more accurately monitor his BP. If I'm doing this under general anesthesia, I would want an EEG monitor if trained personnel are available to interpret the EEG tracings.

Question 5

What other tools could you use to monitor the patient's cerebral function?

Answer 5

Although there is no gold standard for monitoring cerebral function, an awake patient is generally the best guide. If a general technique is used, there are several monitors available, though none of these have been consistently shown to improve outcome: EEG, processed EEG, SSEP, transcranial Doppler, cerebral oximetry, jugular venous oxygen saturation, and stump pressures.

Question 6

If the patient had 90% occlusion of his carotid on the surgical side and 100% occlusion on the other side, which side would you choose for starting the central line if you had to?

Answer 6

If I had to start a central line in this situation, I would prefer to do it on the side with 100% occlusion because if I hit the carotid artery there is no risk of further injury because the vessel is already blocked. Conversely, if I started it on the surgical side and I accidentally punctured the artery, I run the risk of total occlusion of the circulation to the brain, which would be catastrophic in this patient.

Induction

Question 7

How would you induce this patient if you were using a general technique?

Answer 7

My goal in inducing this patient would be to maintain hemodynamic stability, to avoid myocardial ischemia and maintain adequate cerebral perfusion. Thus, assuming the patient has a normal airway, I would use fentanyl, lidocaine, and etomidate. After ensuring that I can ventilate, I would give rocuronium for muscle relaxation and then I would intubate.

Question 8

Immediately after induction, the BP suddenly plummets to 70/40 mmHg. What are you going to do?

Answer 8

I would immediately look at the EKG to make sure this wasn't a malignant rhythm. I would also check the patient's oxygenation and recycle the BP to make sure this was an accurate reading. Assuming all of these parameters were normal, I would open the fluids and give a low-dose vasopressor such as phenylephrine to improve the BP.

Cerebral Ischemia

Question 9

What is meant by "watershed" areas?

Answer 9

"Watershed" areas are those areas of the circulation that lie on the border between the two carotid arteries. Their significance is that during carotid cross-clamp, perfusion from the nonclamped carotid artery needs to be sufficient to prevent a stroke in the patient. However, if the patient has poor perfusion from the nonclamped carotid artery, then there is a high likelihood of a stroke in the "watershed" areas.

Question 10

During placement of the cross-clamp, the EEG technician tells you that there are changes in the EEG waveform. How do you respond?

Answer 10

I would look at my monitors and make sure the patient is not hypoxic, hyper- or hypocarbic, or hypotensive. I would also look at the inhalation agents to make sure the MAC value is less than 0.5. I would then inform the surgeon of these changes and assess if the patient is bleeding profusely, as anemia can also cause such changes. If all of these things were negative, then I would ask the surgeon to release the cross-clamp.

Question 11

The surgeon states he cannot release the cross-clamp at such a crucial part of the procedure. How do you respond?

Answer 11

I would ask him to then place a shunt to allow some blood flow to reach the brain from the carotid artery.

Question 12

Why not place a shunt prophylactically in all patients undergoing this surgery?

Answer 12

Placement of these shunts is not without risks. They can serve as conduits for the movement of small thromboemboli into the neurocirculation and result in life-threatening strokes.

C. Postoperative Care

Postoperative Airway Distress

Question 1

You are paged to the PACU because the nurse says she is noticing a swelling near the surgical site. What are you going to do?

Answer 1

I would go immediately to the patient's bedside and evaluate the patient. I would look at the vital signs to make sure they are stable, evaluate the airway to ensure that there is no airway compromise, make sure the patient is not complaining of stridor or difficulty swallowing, and examine the site of the swelling to see if it is contained or expanding. While notifying the surgeon, I would delineate the margins of the swelling with a marking pen so that I could assess whether the swelling was expanding. If time permitted, I would also send for a CBC and a coagulation profile.

Question 2

The patient develops stridor and complains that he is having some difficulty breathing. How would you respond?

Answer 2

I would immediately place the patient on 100% oxygen via face mask and prepare to emergently intubate the patient at the bedside while calling for help and the difficult-airway cart. I would also look at the surgical site to see if it has continued to expand and have the surgeon paged emergently so we could evacuate any hematoma.

Question 3

Besides a hematoma, what are the other causes of stridor in a postendartectomy patient?

Answer 3

Besides external compression from a hematoma, it could also be from residual anesthetics, such as inadequate reversal of muscle relaxants and inhalation agents, as well as an overdose of postoperative opioid administration.

Postoperative Hypertension

Question 4

During a routine postoperative visit, you notice the BP is 190/100 mmHg. How will you respond?

Answer 4

A malfunctioning carotid sinus is common after these procedures. I would immediately go to the bedside and confirm that this is an accurate reading while assessing the other vital signs to rule out hypoxia, hypercarbia, or a malignant rhythm including myocardial infarction. Next, assuming these were normal, I would try to assess the cause: is the patient anxious or in any discomfort? If no clear etiology could be determined, I would infuse a beta blocker such as labetalol.

Question 5

The surgeon asks if the patient needs to be transferred to the ICU or whether he can be transferred to the general medical floor. How do you respond?

Answer 5

I would want this patient to be transferred to the ICU because this patient is at high risk for hemodynamic instability from the endarterectomy. In addition, given the recent episode of a hematoma in the neck, I would want to watch this patient closely to ensure there is no reaccumulation of blood and that the patient does not develop any more episodes of stridor.

Suggested Readings

Barash PG, Cullen BF, Stoelting RK, Cahalan M, Stock CM, eds. *Clinical Anesthesia*. 6th ed. Philadelphia, PA: Lippincott Williams & Wilkins; 2009.

Ho MD. *The Essential Oral Board Review*. 3rd ed. Houston, TX: Anesthesiology Consultants; 2003.

Thiesen GJ, Grundy BL. Anesthesia and monitoring for carotid endarterectomy. *Bull NY Academy Med*. 1987;63(8):803–819.

29 Cardiovascular: Coronary Artery Bypass Graft (CABG)

Alec C. Runyon and Minh Chau Joe Tran

A 73-year-old, 70 kg female presents to the OR for a three-vessel coronary artery bypass graft (CABG).

History of presenting illness: The patient presented to the ER the day before with complaints of dyspnea and chest pain that she experienced during a hike. Workup revealed a non-ST elevation myocardial infarction (NSTEMI) with subsequent cardiac catheterization, which demonstrated severe three-vessel disease with more than 90% occlusion. The transthoracic echocardiogram (TEE) revealed an ejection fraction (EF) of 25%.

Past medical history: Type 2 diabetes mellitus, hypertension, hypercholesterolemia, COPD with 40 pack-year smoking history (current smoker).

Medications: Hydrochlorothiazide, Metformin, Salmeterol/ Fluticasone inhaler.

Allergies: None.

Physical exam: Vital signs: Pulse = 65 bpm, BP = 105/68 mmHg, RR = 14, O_2 saturation = 92% on RA.

Airway: Mallampati II, full cervical range of motion (ROM), >3 cm thyromental distance.

Lungs: Mildly diminished bilaterally, mild expiratory wheezing.

Cardiovascular: Regular rate, no murmurs.

EKG: Sinus rhythm, HR 65; ST depression in II, III, and aVF; right bundle branch block (RBBB).

Chest X-ray: Hyperinflated lungs, clear, no obvious infiltrates.

Labs: Hb = 14 g/dL, platelets = 250 K, glucose = 190 mg/dL.

A. Preoperative Evaluation

Myocardial Ischemia

Question 1

Describe the pathophysiological differences between an NSTEMI and a STEMI.

Answer 1

The diagnosis of an NSTEMI vs. a STEMI is differentiated by the presence or lack of ST elevations on the EKG. STEMIs are caused by complete blockage of a coronary artery which causes full-thickness ischemia and necrosis to the myocardium. An NSTEMI is caused by partial blockage of the coronary artery which leads to partial-thickness ischemia of the myocardium.

Question 2

How does coronary artery disease (CAD) affect your intraoperative hemodynamic goals for this patient?

Answer 2

In order to prevent myocardial ischemia, there should be an appropriate myocardial oxygen supply and demand balance. Hemodynamic goals should reflect this by maintaining adequate oxygen delivery while minimizing demand via contractility, heart rate, and afterload. Although each anesthetic must be customized to the patient, a general goal is to decrease the heart rate, avoid hypercontractility, and minimize afterload to help decrease myocardial oxygen demand. Hypotension should be avoided to ensure adequate diastolic blood pressure for left coronary artery perfusion.

Question 3

Would you order a stress test?

Answer 3

No, because a stress test would not provide me with any additional information that I do not already have from the catheterization report. In fact, a stress test is an indirect method of measuring coronary ischemia and is not as accurate as a catheterization report. A stress test is routinely obtained because it is noninvasive and so could be done as a first step in screening for CAD. Thus, in light of the latter, the former would not be indicated.

COPD

Question 4

A medical student asks you how this patient's COPD will affect her perioperative course. How would you respond?

Answer 4

Patients with COPD are at increased risk of perioperative pulmonary complications and have an increased postoperative mortality rate. This patient may require a longer postoperative course of mechanical ventilation due to her underlying pulmonary disease. Furthermore, she is more vulnerable to developing pneumonia postoperatively. Intraoperative mechanical ventilation strategies should address her COPD and allow for adequate expiration time.

Diabetes

Question 5

If there is one lab value you could obtain for this patient's diabetes assessment, what value would that be and why?

Answer 5

I would obtain an HbA1C because that gives me an average of blood sugars over the previous 3 months.

B. Intraoperative Management

Monitoring

Question 1

Would you place a pulmonary artery catheter (PAC) in the setting of an RBBB?

Answer 1

I would decide whether the benefits of the PAC outweigh the risks of placement. PAC placement is associated with a small risk of causing new LBBB, which would have deleterious effects in a patient with known RBBB. If I did decide to place the PAC, I would have transcutaneous pacing readily available should a complete heart block develop.

Question 2

Can you use a TEE in place of a PAC?

Answer 2

A TEE certainly has value in determining cardiac output and regional wall motion abnormalities. However, a PAC offers the added benefit of infusing drugs directly into the myocardium, which cannot be done using a TEE.

Induction

Question 3

What medications would you use to induce general anesthesia for this patient and why?

Answer 3

My goals would be to induce anesthesia while maintaining hemodynamic stability. Thus, after preoxygenation with 100% oxygen, assuming a normal airway, I would induce with fentanyl, lidocaine, etomidate, and, after ensuring ventilation, rocuronium.

Question 4

Are you concerned about the adrenal suppression that often accompanies etomidate?

Answer 4

Although etomidate has been associated with adrenal suppression, this usually occurs with repeat boluses or an infusion. The benefits of a smooth induction in a patient with severe CAD and systolic heart failure outweigh the potential risks for this patient.

Question 5

After a successful intubation, the patient's heart rate climbs to the 130s and you notice slight worsening of her ST depressions. What would you do next?

Answer 5

I would immediately put the patient on 100% oxygen and look at the other vital signs, making sure the patient is not hypoxic, hypercarbic, hypotensive, or in a malignant arrhythmia. Assuming adequate oxygenation, ventilation, and blood pressure, I would administer a beta blocker such as esmolol to reduce myocardial demand while maintaining normotension.

Bypass Considerations

Question 6

The patient's blood pressure increases to 165/95 at the time of aortic cannulation. Is this concerning and if so, why?

Answer 6

Yes, because hypertension during aortic cannulation can be problematic because of the increased risk of aortic dissection. Ideally, blood pressure should be in the low–normal range to decrease this risk. Methods to assess for a dissection include evaluating pump flows and pressures, observing blood pressure correlation between the cannula and a peripheral arterial line, aortic pressure waveform analysis, and TEE imaging of the cannula and aorta.

Question 7

Your medical student asks how you are sure that anesthesia is maintained during cardiopulmonary bypass (CPB) now that your ventilator and anesthetic is off. How do you respond?

Answer 7

During CPB, the perfusionist administers volatile anesthetics through their bypass machine. The anesthesiologist should verify that this task is not forgotten so that amnesia and anesthesia are maintained. Furthermore, the hypothermia used during CPB decreases awareness and MAC, aiding in the anesthetic. During rewarming, however, cerebral temperatures increase faster than core temperatures, which places the patient at increased risk of intraoperative awareness. I would administer midazolam as we rewarm the patient to minimize the risk of awareness. I would also use a BIS monitor throughout the case to aid my decision-making.

Question 8

Describe what steps you would take to wean the patient off of cardiopulmonary bypass.

Answer 8

I would begin by rewarming the patient to normothermia and administering midazolam to minimize the risk of intraoperative awareness. I would turn on all alarms and monitors that may have been turned off or silenced when going on CPB. I would suction the endotracheal tube and then initiate ventilation when appropriate. I would verify that my intravenous lines are still functioning and that any potential infusions or pressors are prepared. I would correct any laboratory abnormalities and call for blood products to the room if there is concern for post-bypass bleeding. I would also evaluate the cardiac function of the heart using vital signs, pressure waveforms, and echocardiographic evaluation of the heart. I would make sure the heart is deaired and would work closely with the surgical team to come off bypass at the appropriate time. I would ensure that volatile anesthetic agent continues to be delivered to the patient via the anesthesia machine after separation from bypass.

Coagulation

Question 9

With the goal of minimizing perioperative bleeding, you administered aminocaproic acid after the initial incision. What is the mechanism of action of aminocaproic acid?

Answer 9

Aminocaproic acid is a lysine analog that binds to plasminogen and plasmin, interfering with fibrinolysis, thus decreasing bleeding.

Question 10

After cardiopulmonary bypass, the surgeon states that there is diffuse bleeding in the operative field and the patient does not seem to be clotting normally. What factors predict post-bypass bleeding?

Answer 10

The bypass machine can induce a coagulopathy by hemodilution, systemic inflammatory response syndrome (SIRS) activation, causing platelets to stick to the bypass circuit, and contact activation of the coagulation pathway. Other predictors of bleeding after bypass including preoperative hemoglobin and platelet levels, recent history of anticoagulant and/or antiplatelet use, and CPB time. Additionally, surgical causes of bleeding should also be evaluated.

C. Postoperative Care

ICU Transfer of Care

Question 1

You take the patient to the ICU intubated. The ICU team asks you if this patient is a candidate for early extubation. How would you respond?

Answer 1

The timing of postoperative extubation is multifactorial. It depends on the course of the surgery, current hemodynamic and laboratory status, and patient comorbidities. This patient has a history of COPD with low SpO2 at baseline. This may prolong postoperative extubation. Additionally, if there were intraoperative complications, this may further prolong the time for extubation.

Question 2

As you are preparing to leave the room after transferring care to the ICU team, the bedside nurse tells you that the patient went from normal sinus rhythm to supraventricular tachycardia (SVT) on the monitor. What would you do?

Answer 2

I would immediately assess the other vital signs and confirm adequate ventilation and oxygenation. I would then confirm that the rhythm was, in fact, SVT. I would check blood pressure and verify that the patient has a pulse. In accordance with the American College of Cardiology/American Heart Association (ACC/AHA) guidelines for tachycardia with a pulse, I would then evaluate for hypotension, altered mental status, or other signs suggestive of ischemia and/or acute heart failure. If any of these issues were found, I would consider synchronized cardioversion with 50–100 J. If the patient was otherwise stable, I would obtain an EKG and consider vagal maneuvers and adenosine if the patient was regular and monomorphic. I would also consider esmolol and fluid administration depending on the clinical picture.

Postoperative Management

Question 3

A postoperative hemoglobin is 7.5 g/dL. Vital signs and other labs are normal. Would you transfuse?

Answer 3

The decision to transfuse depends on several factors, including current vital signs, patient comorbidities, recent fluid status and blood loss, and perioperative course, among others. If this patient's vital signs appeared within normal range and there were no other significant metabolic derangements or lab abnormalities, I would choose a restrictive transfusion strategy and monitor the patient's course.

Question 4

What are the risks of blood transfusions?

Answer 4

Risks of blood transfusions include hemolytic and nonhemolytic reactions, transmission of infectious diseases, febrile reactions, and allergic reactions.

Hyperglycemia

Question 5

The postoperative labs reveal a blood sugar of 240 mg/dL. What are the risks of hyperglycemia in the perioperative period?

Answer 5

Hyperglycemia is associated with slower wound healing and increased rates of surgical site infections, myocardial infarctions, stroke, and death. Hyperglycemia can also lead to increased postoperative complications and prolonged hospital courses.

Suggested Reading

Barash PG, Cullen BF, Stoelting RK, Cahalan M, Stock CM, eds. *Clinical Anesthesia*. 6th ed. Philadelphia, PA: Lippincott Williams & Wilkins; 2009.

30 Cardiovascular: Abdominal Aortic Aneurysm

Carl Ying and Minh Chau Joe Tran

A 58-year-old male is scheduled for repair of a 6.5 cm abdominal aortic aneurysm (AAA) that was discovered during routine checkup.

Past medical history: DM 2, HTN, CAD, and COPD. The patient reports a 40 pack-year smoking history and metabolic equivalents (METS) >4.

Vital signs: BP 130/87 mmHg, HR 72 bpm, RR 13 breaths, saturation 93% on RA.

Physical exam: Unremarkable airway and physical exam. He is comfortable in the preoperative area and is without any complaints.

Chest X-ray shows mild hyperinflation.

The patient has a recent CBC and metabolic panel significant for Hgb 10.1 and Cr 1.4. HbA1C is 7.6. EKG shows NSR.

Echocardiogram: 5 months ago it showed an EF of 65% without major valvular dysfunction.

A. Preoperative Evaluation

Question 1

What medications should a typical AAA patient take the day of surgery?

Answer 1

The patient should continue his beta blockers, statins, and usually ASA as well. Diuretics and angiotensin-converting enzyme (ACE) inhibitors should be considered on a case-by-case basis. If the patient is taking Plavix and other antiplatelet agents, especially if needed for a stent, I would need to have a discussion with the cardiologist who prescribed it.

Question 2

How would you evaluate this patient's cardiac status?

Answer 2

Before I ordered any tests, I would conduct a history and physical. From the history, I would evaluate the patient's cardiac status by asking about baseline exercise level, any recent history of chest pain, and any recent changes in his medications. From the physical exam I would look at the vital signs, specifically the heart rate, to evaluate if the patient is effectively beta blocked. I would also evaluate for signs of heart failure, such as JVD, pedal edema, or pulmonary edema. Lastly, I would look at the baseline EKG.

Question 3

Would you want any pulmonary function tests for this patient?

Answer 3

No. PFTs would not provide me with any additional information beyond what a thorough history and physical would.

Question 4

What are your anesthetic and hemodynamic goals for this surgery?

Answer 4

My goal is to maintain organ perfusion, intravascular volume, and carefully control BP to prevent rupture of aneurysm. To that end, I would aim for a BP within 20% of this patient's baseline.

B. Intraoperative Management

Question 1

What monitors and equipment would you prepare for this patient?

Answer 1

In addition to standard ASA monitors, I would want to monitor arterial/venous pressure as well as urine output. I would plan for an A-line prior to induction and central venous line after intubation. I would consider cardiac output monitoring and TEE in select patients, or if this patient becomes unstable. PAC monitoring is controversial but may be useful in patients with additional cardiac comorbidities.

Question 2

What is your plan for induction and maintenance?

Answer 2

Since this is an open procedure, I would opt for a slow, controlled induction using fentanyl, lidocaine, etomidate, and rocuronium.

For maintenance, I would use a balanced anesthetic technique with volatile anesthetics combined with opiates and a thoracic epidural (placed preoperatively). I would plan to load the thoracic epidural after unclamping and after hemodynamics had stabilized.

Question 3

What should you expect to happen during aortic clamping and how would you manage it?

Answer 3

During clamping, I would expect increased arterial pressure, increased afterload, and increased left ventricular end diastolic wall stress, the degree of which depends on the position of clamp. Ejection fraction and cardiac output may decrease, and ischemia or heart failure may occur. To manage the hypertensive response, I could increase anesthetic depth or use short-acting beta blockers or short-acting vasodilators, such as nitroglycerin or sodium nitroprusside.

Question 4

What should you expect to happen during unclamping and how would you manage it?

Answer 4

During unclamping, I would expect hypotension due to the significant decrease in SVR, release of cytokines and metabolites from ischemic tissues, and hypovolemia from redistribution of blood to the reperfused tissues. Generally, longer clamp time and more cephalad clamps result in worse hypotension. I would administer fluids before clamp removal and have vasopressors and/or inotropes available to stabilize the blood pressure. Even if not needed during clamping, I might use vasodilators to allow additional fluid loading, to raise filling pressures to slightly above normal. I would also make prophylactic ventilator adjustments to account for increased acidic load from ischemic tissue. It is important to communicate with the surgeon to prepare for the hemodynamic changes that come with removal of the clamp.

Question 5

After the surgeon releases the clamp, the BP drops despite aggressive fluid and vasopressor administration. What is your next step?

Answer 5

I would ask the surgeon to reapply the aortic cross-clamp in order to stabilize the patient. I would ensure adequate fluid resuscitation (with the goal CVP of 12–15 mmHg) and attempt to unclamp again slowly. I would also check to make sure all vasodilators were off and vasopressors/inotropes were on.

My differential diagnosis would also include hemorrhage and MI/heart failure. I would use a TEE to further evaluate this patient if he did not tolerate unclamping after optimization.

Question 6

How would your anesthetic plan change if this was an endovascular repair?

Answer 6

While general anesthesia is certainly an option, neuraxial techniques can also be considered in certain populations. Neuraxial techniques have been shown to have reduced cardiopulmonary complications and shorter ICU/hospital length of stay. However, I would still be prepared to convert to a general anesthetic as the case may be converted to an open procedure at any time.

C. Postoperative Care

Question 1

You notice the patient's blood pressure is 85/54 mmHg with a HR of 65 bpm in the PACU. What do you do?

Answer 1

I would examine the patient at the bedside. I would make sure the patient is not hypoxic and is adequately ventilating. If the EKG and other vital signs were normal, I would check the patient's hemoglobin and evaluate the fluid status. I would provide fluids or blood as necessary.

Question 2

The PACU nurse asks you, "Since this case involves an infrarenal aneurysm, his kidneys should be fine, right?" What strategies can you use to protect renal function?

Answer 2

Even when the clamp is placed distal to the renal arteries, decreased renal function is a common complication. Renal complications after AAA surgery are due to a decrease in blood flow with an increase in renal vascular resistance. Myoglobin release from ischemic tissues may cause acute tubular necrosis (ATN).

The key is prevention with optimization of volume and hemodynamics. Diuretics are often considered after adequate resuscitation. Low-dose dopamine may improve renal blood flow and urine output but has not been proven to decrease postoperative renal failure. Mannitol can be used for renal protection.

Question 3

The PACU nurse calls you in 30 minutes to inform you that the patient is reporting he cannot move his legs in the PACU. What is your differential diagnosis?

Answer 3

My first concern would be spinal cord ischemia. The anterior spinal artery is supplied by multiple segmental arteries. Spinal cord ischemia can occur from decreased blood flow through these critical segmental arteries and hypotension distal to the clamp.

A key segmental artery is the artery of Adamkiewicz. It arises from a branch from a left intercostal artery between T9 and T12 in 75% of the population and is critical to the blood supply of the anterior spinal artery. Interference with this artery is often the cause of paraplegia.

Also on my differential list is a thromboembolic phenomenon and a compressive lesion (MRI should be done immediately, as this may be curable). EMG studies may indicate the site of the lesion and help with the prognosis.

Question 4

What other complications are common after this surgery?

Answer 4

Cardiovascular: MI, dysrhythmias (15%)

Respiratory: Pneumonia, atelectasis, respiratory failure, and PE (10%)

Renal complications: Acute kidney injury, ATN, dialysis (2–5%)

GI: Bowel ischemia, acute abdomen and compartment syndrome (3–4%)

Hemorrhage (2–4%)

Neurological: Cerebrovascular disease, cognitive dysfunction, confusion/delirium, paraplegia

Surgical: leg ischemia, infection, hernia, deep venous thrombosis (DVT)/PEs

Suggested Readings

Al-Hashimi M, Thompson J. Anaesthesia for elective open abdominal aortic aneurysm repair. *Continuing Educ Anaesth Crit Care Pain.* 2013; 13(6):208–212.

Barash PG, Cullen BF, Stoelting R, eds. *Clinical Anesthesia.* 6th ed. Philadelphia, PA: Lippincott Williams & Wilkins; 2009: 1122–1132

Jaffe R. *Anesthesiologists Manual of Surgical Procedures.* Philadelphia, PA: Lippincott Williams & Wilkins; 2014.

31 Obstetric: Hemorrhage

Edouard Belotte

A 32-year-old G2P1 with twin gestation presents to the obstetric floor for vaginal bleeding.

History of present illness: Her previous pregnancy resulted in a cesarean section, but she had hoped for a vaginal delivery this time for her 36-week gestational twins.

Past medical history: Gestational diabetes, COPD.

Smoking history: 10 pack-year smoker, did not smoke during pregnancy.

Physical exam: Vital signs: pulse = 87 bpm, RR = 18, BP = 120/76 mmHg, O_2 = 97% on RA.

Airway: Mallampati III, full cervical range of motion.

Cardiovascular: Regular rate and rhythm.

Pulmonary: Clear to auscultation.

Labs: Hb = 9.1 g/dL, platelets = 240 K, WBC = 12.1 K/uL, Na = 138 mEq/L, K = 4.5 mEq/L.

A. Preoperative Evaluation

Hemodynamics

Question 1

How would you assess this patient's hemodynamic status?

Answer 1

I would go to the patient's bedside and perform a history and physical. From the history I would ask the patient about any complaints of lightheadedness, nausea, positional vertigo, or syncopal episodes. From the physical exam, I would look at her vital signs, especially the blood pressure and heart rate to evaluate for hypotension and reflex tachycardia. I could also look for signs of hypovolemia, such as capillary refill time, moisture of mucous membranes, and skin turgor to determine if this patient's blood loss has resulted in hypovolemia with progression to hemodynamic instability.

Bleeding Etiology

Question 2

What is the differential diagnosis of third-trimester bleeding?

Answer 2

The most common causes of third-trimester hemorrhage are placenta previa and placental abruption. Placenta previa is the abnormal implantation of the placenta in front of the fetal presenting part. Placental abruption is separation of the placenta from the decidua basalis before delivery of the fetus. There is a strong association between a previous uterine scar and the development of placenta previa.

Less common causes of antepartum hemorrhage are cervical pathology such as polyps carcinoma, uterine rupture, vasa previa, and local genital tract lesions. Pre-eclampsia and intrauterine death place patients at risk for coagulopathies, which may give rise to maternal hemorrhage.

Question 3

How do you distinguish a placenta previa from a placenta abruption?

Answer 3

The definitive diagnosis of each is determined by ultrasound, but a focused history can often help make the distinction. A placenta previa will present with painless vaginal bleeding, whereas placenta abruption will present with painful bleeding.

Question 4

What are the most common clinical manifestations of each?

Answer 4

Patients with placenta previa have painless, bright red vaginal bleeding that rarely progresses to hypovolemic shock and disseminated intravascular coagulation (DIC), and patients with placental abruption have port-wine nonclotted, painful bleeding that commonly progresses to hypovolemic shock and DIC.

Double Setup

Question 5

What is a double setup? When it is indicated?

Answer 5

A double setup is a vaginal examination performed in the OR with the immediate capability of converting to cesarean section under general anesthesia. It is indicated whenever there is a real chance of needing to convert rapidly to general anesthesia. The entire obstetric team needs to be present (anesthesiologist, obstetrician, pediatrician, nurse, and surgical technician).

The patient should have large-bore intravenous access, standard monitoring, and appropriate anesthetic drugs available in the OR.

Uterine Rupture

Question 6

Who is at risk for uterine rupture? How is uterine rupture diagnosed?

Answer 6

Uterine rupture is a potentially life-threatening condition that occurs in patients with previous uterine scars such as those from a cesarean section. Risk factors include use of prostaglandins, uterine trauma, a tumultuous labor, midforceps delivery, breech version and extraction, inappropriate uterotonic use, uterine anomalies, placenta percreta, tumors, fetal macrosomia, and fetal malposition. The most consistent sign of uterine rupture is fetal distress. Other signs that may be present include hypotension, vaginal bleeding, abdominal pain, change in the uterine contour, changes in the uterine contraction pattern, and cessation of labor. True diagnosis is made either during manual inspection of the uterus or during a laparotomy.

Preoperative Labs

Question 7

Do you want any additional laboratory assessments done before taking this patient to the operating room?

Answer 7

Yes. I would order a coagulation profile (to determine suitability for neuraxial technique as well as an early indicator for DIC) and type and cross for two units of PRBC.

B. Intraoperative Management

Regional vs. General

Question 1

Would you use a regional or a general anesthetic for this patient?

Answer 1

Based on the information given, this patient is currently hemodynamically stable. If her bleeding was not brisk and her overall blood loss not significant, I would want to perform an epidural in this patient. If, however, she displayed any signs of hypovolemia or she was actively hemorrhaging I would want to avoid the sympathectomy caused by the epidural and instead opt to do this case under general anesthesia.

Monitoring

Question 2

What invasive monitors, if any, would you place?

Answer 2

I would place a radial arterial line to detect any abrupt changes in blood pressure and to allow access for blood sampling for serial hematocrit, ABG, and coagulation in the event the patient's condition deteriorates. I would also ensure that a Foley catheter is placed to assess adequacy of urine output. Finally, if I didn't have at least two 18 g PIVs or better, I would place a central line.

Transfusion

Question 3

Would you transfuse blood to this patient before administering anesthesia?

Answer 3

Transfusion of blood products should be guided by the volume of blood loss over time and changes in hemodynamic parameters (e.g., blood pressure, maternal and fetal heart rates, peripheral perfusion, and urine output) as well as the hemoglobin level. Thus, assuming the patient was otherwise stable with reassuring fetal heart rate (FHR) tracing, I would not rush to transfusion.

Induction

Question 4

Assuming a general anesthetic technique is selected, how would you induce this patient for the cesarean section?

Answer 4

Because this patient is considered to have a full stomach, I would premedicate with sodium citrate before induction of general anesthesia. After preoxygenation with 100% oxygen, I would perform a rapid sequence induction with cricoid pressure using fentanyl, etomidate, and succinylcholine.

Intraoperative Hemorrhage

Question 5

The patient is hemorrhaging after removal of the placenta. Her blood pressure reads 95/50 mmHg. Heart rate is 106 bpm and oxygen saturation is 96%. What is your management?

Answer 5

While recycling the blood pressure, I would open fluids wide open, place the patient in the Trendelenburg position with head down, and administer a small dose of phenylephrine. I would concurrently communicate with the surgeon to determine if the hemorrhage is ongoing. If it is and the patient continues to be hypotensive, I would immediately begin the blood transfusion.

Question 6

How would you assess for the amount of blood loss?

Answer 6

Blood loss needs to be assessed by looking at the operating field, communicating with the surgeon, counting the sponges soaked, and checking the suction canister.

Question 7

What is the role of cell salvage in obstetric patients?

Answer 7

The use of intraoperative cell salvage for peripartum hemorrhage is still controversial, although major obstetric anesthesia societies now regard it as an acceptable alternative to allogeneic transfusion. The fear is that amniotic fluid components will be administered to the patient and cause an amniotic fluid embolism. However, intraoperative cell salvage has been shown to have an undisputed role in obstetric patients with high risk such as placenta previa/accreta, massive fibroids, or rare blood type or unusual antibodies. Intraoperative cell salvage can be also useful in the treatment of Jehovah's Witnesses. Cell saver may decrease the risk of blood-borne infections associated with transfusion of banked red blood cells (RBCs) and may also decrease the risk of alloimmunization. The risks of transfusion reactions and transfusion-related acute lung injury would also be reduced if autologous blood was used instead of banked blood.

Question 8

What invasive options are available to control peripartum hemorrhage (PPH) when medical treatment is unsuccessful to control the bleeding?

Answer 8

Several invasive options are available to control PPH when medical treatments fail:

Uterine balloon tamponade: Uterine packing has long been the treatment of choice to manage PPH; it is safe, quick, and easily performed by relatively inexperienced personnel and can be performed with or without anesthesia.

Uterine arterial embolization: It has become a well-recognized alternative method of treatment in the conservative management of PPH in association with local or medical treatment, or in the event of their failure. This therapeutic approach avoids morbidity associated with peripartum hysterectomy and preserves fertility. It is also a possible additional approach when arterial ligation or hysterectomy fails to control bleeding.

Surgical iliac (or uterine) artery ligation: When uterine tamponade and arterial embolization fail, a laparotomy to perform iliac artery ligation is an option to preserve the uterus. It can also be performed as a first invasive option, during cesarean section delivery, or when the patient is hemodynamically unstable or if embolization is not readily available.

B-Lynch suture: Since its first description in 1997, the so-called B-Lynch uterine compression suture has been used successfully to control bleeding following failed conservative management.

Emergency hysterectomy may be required to control bleeding refractory to other methods and to save lives.

C. Postoperative Management

Postpartum Hemorrhage

Question 1

The patient is now in the PACU after the cesarean section. You are called to see this patient because of continuing hemorrhage. What is the definition of postpartum hemorrhage?

Answer 1

PPH is defined as blood loss of more than 500 mL following vaginal delivery or more than 1000 mL following cesarean delivery. A loss of these amounts within 24 hours of delivery is termed early or primary PPH, whereas such losses are termed late or secondary PPH if they occur 24 hours after delivery. Another proposal suggests using a 10% fall in hematocrit value to define PPH. Patients with unexplained hypotension, tachycardia, or low urine output should be suspected as having a PPH, and resuscitation should commence.

Question 2

What is the differential diagnosis of PPH?

Answer 2

PPH has many potential causes, but the most common is uterine atony (failure of the uterus to contract and retract upon delivery of the baby). Other risk factors are high birthweight, labor induction and augmentation, chorioamnionitis, magnesium sulfate use, previous PPH, and uterine causes such as retained products of conception, placental accreta, uterine inversion, and uterine rupture. Nonuterine causes include genital tract lesions, genital tract hematomas, intra-abdominal lacerations, pelvic lacerations, and coagulopathies, including DIC.

Question 3

How will you assess this patient with PPH?

HEMORRHAGE

Answer 3

I would go immediately to the bedside and perform a focused history and physical. From the history, I would review the chart to see how much blood loss has occurred intraoperatively and postoperatively. I would also look to see what fluids, pressors, and blood products she received during this time. I would ask the patient if she feels light-headed or nauseous and whether there is any change in her mentation. I would also look at how much urine output she has had. From the physical, I would first look at her vital signs to evaluate for hypotension and tachycardia. I would see if she is still bleeding and look for any bloody sheets or towels. Finally, I would look for any signs of DIC (widespread bruising or hemorrhage) and order a stat CBC, coagulation, and d-dimer and inform the surgeon.

Suggested Readings

Blomberg M. Maternal obesity and risk of postpartum hemorrhage. *Obstet Gynecol.* 2011;118(3):561–568.

Clark SL, Koonings PP, Phelan JP. Placenta previa/accreta and prior cesarean section. *Obstet Gynecol.* 1985;66(1):89–92.

Gabbe SG, Niebyl JR, Galan HL, Jauniaux ER, Landon MB, et al. *Gabbe: Obstetrics: Normal and Problem Pregnancies.* 6th ed. Philadelphia: PA. Elsevier Saunders; 2012.

Jackson KW Jr, Allbert JR, Schemmer GK, Elliot M, Humphrey A, Taylor J. A randomized controlled trial comparing oxytocin administration before and after placental delivery in the prevention of postpartum hemorrhage. *Am J Obstet Gynecol.* 2001;185(4):873–877

Mayer DC, Spielman FJ, Bell EA. Antepartum and postpartum hemorrhage. In: Chestnut DH, ed. *Obstetric Anesthesia: Principles and Practice.* 3rd ed. St. Louis, MO: Mosby, 2004: 668–671.

Wali A, Suresh MS, Gregg AR. Antepartum hemorrhage. In: Datta S, ed. *Anesthetic and Obstetric Management of High-Risk Pregnancy.* 3rd ed. New York: Springer; 2004: 94–98.

32 Obstetric: Preeclampsia

Xiaodong Bao

Stem 2

A 23-year-old, 85 kg, G3P1 female who is 36 weeks pregnant is admitted to labor and delivery (L&D) for an urgent cesarean section due to premature rupture of membrane. She has had very limited prenatal care and is not on any regular medications. Her past medical history is significant for chronic intravenous drug abuse (IVDA). On admission, her vital signs are BP 150/110 mmHg, HR 100 bpm, SaO_2 96% on RA. Hb is 10.1 g/dL.

A. Preoperative Evaluation

Drug Abuse

Question 1

What are your anesthetic concerns regarding this patient?

Answer 1

I have concerns for both the mother and fetus. Regarding the mother, I am concerned about her IVDA status. She could have poor IV access, may have used multiple kinds of drugs, have increased risk of diseases such as hepatitis and HIV, and have drug dependence and withdrawal syndrome, and systemic derangement depending on the drugs used. I am also worried about her limited prenatal care, which predisposes both mother and fetus to much higher peripartum complications. She may have undiagnosed preeclampsia, as evidenced by her high blood pressure. Uncontrolled hypertension and cocaine abuse substantially increases the risk of placenta abruption. There is also an increased chance of postpartum hemorrhage. Regarding the fetus, I am concerned that the baby may suffer intrauterine growth restriction (IUGR), intraventricular hemorrhage, congenital abnormalities, and low birth weight. The fetus could have had sustained exposure to various abusive drugs that results in fetal dependence and withdrawal syndrome.

Question 2

What are your differential diagnoses for hypertension in this patient?

Answer 2

There are abundant reasons for this patient being hypertensive. She may have untreated chronic hypertension, gestational hypertension, preeclampsia, or drug-induced hypertension, such as from cocaine or amphetamines.

Question 3

The patient adamantly denies having any medical problems before pregnancy. She reluctantly admits that she does use cocaine frequently. Do you think the patient's elevated blood pressure is due to the cocaine use? How would you differentiate that from baseline preeclampsia?

Answer 3

Cocaine use can certainly lead to sympathetic activation with maternal hypertension, tachycardia, arrhythmia, and myocardial ischemia. In severe cases, hyperreflexia and convulsions due to cocaine abuse can mimic preeclampsia/eclampsia. I would obtain a more detailed history and physical, including routes of administration, last time of drug use, amount taken, duration of use, and medical treatments she has undergone. I would also look for signs of cocaine use such as dilated pupils, increased heart rate, arrhythmia, and agitation. I would send for a toxicology screen as well as urinalysis to help me determine the cause of her high blood pressure.

Question 4

The urine test comes back negative for cocaine. What does this mean?

Answer 4

It means that the patient probably has not used cocaine in the last 3–5 days.

Preeclampsia

Question 5

What is preeclampsia? How is that distinguished from severe preeclampsia?

Answer 5

Preeclampsia is a multiorgan disorder that presents after 20 weeks' gestation with remission usually by 48 hours after delivery. It is characterized by sustained systolic blood pressure (SBP) of at least 140 mmHg or diastolic blood pressure (DBP) of at least 90 mmHg (more than twice, 4 to 6 hours apart) and proteinuria with ≥300 mg protein in 24-hour urine collection.

Severe preeclampsia is diagnosed if there is preeclampsia plus one of following:

- Sustained SBP ≥160 mmHg or DBP ≥110 mmHg
- Evidence of end-organ damage
- Deteriorating renal function, including severe proteinuria (>5 g/24 hr), sudden oliguria, especially with elevated creatinine
- CNS disturbance (headache, vision disturbance)

- Liver dysfunction
- Thrombocytopenia
- HELLP syndrome
- Epigastric/right upper quadrant pain (stretching of hepatic capsule)
- Pulmonary edema
- Fetal compromise (IUGR, oligohydramnios, nonreassuring fetal testing)

Question 6

You suspect that the patient has preeclampsia. What laboratory test(s) would you order?

Answer 6

I would send for a CBC, BMP, liver function test to assess for HELLP syndrome, uric acid test, urinalysis, 24-hour urine protein, and a coagulation study.

B. Intraoperative Management

Magnesium Therapy

Question 1

Should you stop the magnesium infusion before the procedure?

Answer 1

No. Magnesium sulfate is first-line drug treatment for seizure prophylaxis.

Question 2

What are the pharmacodynamic effects of magnesium sulfate?

Answer 2

Magnesium sulfate decreases the release of acetylcholine and decreases the sensitivity of the motor endplate to acetylcholine. It has following effects (with *VAST* as their mnemonic):

- **V**: vasodilation-hypotension
- **A**: anticonvulsant
- **S**: sedative, skeletal muscle relaxant; increased sensitivity to both depolarizing and nondepolarizing muscle relaxants. Fasciculation may not be observed after succinylcholine.
- **T**: tocolytic (decreases uterine activity), which increases uterine blood flow

Question 3

What are the side effects of magnesium sulfate?

Answer 3

- Diminished deep tendon reflexes (4–5 mEq/L)
- EKG changes, including prolonged PR and ST intervals, widened QRS complexes, and/or elevated T waves (4–7 mEq/L)
- Somnolence (5–7 mEq/L)
- Loss of deep tendon reflexes, or myotonia (8–10 mEq/L)
- Heart block (12 mEq/L)
- Respiratory arrest (15 mEq/L)
- Cardiac arrest and cardiovascular collapse (20 mEq/L)

Thrombocytopenia

Question 4

The platelet number comes back at 90 K. Are you comfortable with placing an epidural for this case?

Answer 4

Yes, as long as this is a steady-state platelet count and there has been no recent abrupt decline. A common rule of thumb is that if the platelet count is >75 K, in the absence of other coagulation abnormalities, one would not expect to see an increased likelihood of neuraxial anesthetic complications in the setting of preeclampsia.

Question 5

If there are no previous labs studies on this patient, would you still proceed with an epidural technique, with a platelet number of 75 K?

Answer 5

Although I would be very concerned by this level, I would still proceed with an epidural technique, as long as the patient does not demonstrate increased bleeding tendencies on the history and physical exam. The obstetricians and patient would need to be counseled on the risks and benefits of the procedure before obtaining consent from the patient. Blood products including platelets should be in the room prior to starting surgery.

Deceleration

Question 6

Before performing the epidural, there is an episode of late deceleration on the FHR monitor, and the obstetrician decides on a stat Cesarean section. How would this change your anesthetic plan?

Answer 6

I would perform a single-shot spinal for the stat cesarean section. Traditionally, spinal anesthesia has been avoided for inducing when there is a dramatic swing in blood pressure in preeclamptic patients. More recent studies demonstrate that single-shot spinal, combined-spinal epidural, and epidural anesthesia can all be used effectively for this patient population. In some studies, because of vasoconstriction, incidence and severity of hypotension after single-shot spinal are less in women with preeclampsia than in healthy women. In this patient, I would use a spinal anesthetic because it provides a denser surgical block, and we can administer intrathecal narcotics for better postoperative pain control. In addition, the fetus is already presenting with distress. A spinal anesthetic has a faster onset, which can save valuable time for the fetus.

Question 7

After 5 minutes of successfully placing the spinal anesthetic, the patient's BP plummets to 60/40 mmHg and she begins to complain of severe nausea. How do you respond?

Answer 7

I would immediately place the patient in the left uterine displacement position, give supplemental oxygen, open the fluids wide, assess the dermatomal level, check the FHR, and begin boluses of pressors such as phenylephrine or ephedrine.

Induction

Question 8

That issue is now resolved. As the surgeon begins to "test" the abdomen for sensation, the patient begins to scream loudly, complaining that she feels everything. If your decision is to convert to a general anesthetic, how would you induce the patient?

Answer 8

After preoxygenation with 100% oxygen and administering Bicitra and metoclopramide, I would perform an RSI with cricoid pressure using fentanyl, lidocaine, propofol, and succinylcholine, assuming she has a normal-appearing airway.

C. Postoperative Care

Postpartum Hemorrhage

Question 1

The cesarean section was uneventful and you extubate the patient in the OR. You are now paged by the PACU nurse because the patient has abnormal vaginal bleeding. What will you do?

Answer 1

I would go immediately to the bedside and assess the patient. I would check the vital signs, urine output, mental status, acuity of blood loss, and quantify the blood loss by counting the number of soaked vaginal pads. After informing the obstetrician, I would establish large-bore IVs to support the blood pressure with crystalloids and phenylephrine, call for four units of PRBCs, send a stat CBC to determine the Hb level, and have a colleague prepare the OR for possible re-exploration.

Question 2

If the bleeding is caused by uterine atony, how would you manage this?

Answer 2

First, I would actively resuscitate the patient by placing her on 100% oxygen and opening the IV fluids. Second, I would carefully review the chart to see if the patient received or is receiving any offending agents that should be stopped immediately. I would give the patient a second dose of oxytocin and consider using Hemabate. I would avoid using ergot alkaloids because of the risk of a hypertensive crisis.

Seizure

Question 3

This issue is resolved. A few hours later you are paged to the PACU because the patient has developed a seizure. Why did this happen?

Answer 3

The risk of a preeclamptic patient developing seizures remains 24–48 hours after delivery. Thus the patient needs to be maintained on magnesium therapy.

Postoperative Hypotension

Question 4

On POD #1 you notice that her BP has been reading approximately 75/50 mmHg. Why do you think this is happening?

Answer 4

There are several potential causes of hypotension in this patient. She could be hypoxic, hypocarbic, or in a malignant arrhythmia. She may also be volume depleted secondary to her delivery and perhaps needs more IV fluids or PO fluids, if tolerated. She still may also be bleeding, with resultant anemia and hypotension. Finally, her magnesium therapy, which should still be ongoing, has hypotensive side effects.

Suggested Readings

Crosby ET. Obstetrical anaesthesia for patients with the syndrome of haemolysis, elevated liver enzymes and low platelets. *Can J Anaesth*. 1991;38 (2):227–233.

Dennis AT. Management of pre-eclampsia: issues for anaesthetists. *Anaesthesia.* 2012;67(9):1009–1020.
Mercier FJ. Cesarean delivery fluid management. *Curr Opin Anaesthesiol.* 2012;25(3):286–291.
Turner JA. Diagnosis and management of pre-eclampsia: an update. *Int J Womens Health.* 2010;30(2):327–337.

33 Additional Topics: Cardiac

Ruchir Gupta

Heparin

1. A 56-year-old male is undergoing an on-pump coronary artery bypass graft (CABG) procedure for four-vessel disease.

Question 1a

How do you determine how much heparin to administer?

Answer 1a

The initial dose of heparin is 3–4 mg/kg. I would begin with this dose and then check an activated clotting time (ACT) to determine if I had reached the therapeutic goal of 300–400 seconds. If I had not achieved that level, I would administer additional heparin.

Question 1b

What are some adverse effects of protamine?

Answer 1b

Protamine can cause hypotension, anaphylaxis, pulmonary hypertension, and anaphylactoid reactions.

Cardiac Tamponade

2. You are paged to the ICU because a 75-year-old patient, post–aortic valve replacement, has had a steady decrease in BP. His current vital signs are BP = 101/80 mmHg, HR = 85 bmp, RR = 14, O_2 saturation 98% on 40% FiO_2. A bedside echocardiogram reveals a cardiac tamponade.

Question 2a

What is Beck's triad?

Answer 2a

Beck's triad is jugular venous distension, hypotension, and muffled heart sounds.

Question 2b

The patient is rushed to the OR for an emergent pericardial window. Assuming the patient was extubated prior to this event, what would be your goals during induction? How do you plan on achieving them?

Answer 2b

Initially, I would advocate for performing a pericardiocentesis under local anesthesia, to relieve some of the tamponade before induction and improve hemodynamics. If this is not possible, my goals during induction would be to maintain cardiac output, spontaneous ventilation, and blood pressure. With a preinduction A-line in place, I would administer midazolam and ketamine, because ketamine will increase myocardial contractility, systemic vascular resistance, and heart rate. Once the pericardial sac is opened and drained, I would administer rocuronium.

Hypertrophic Cardiomyopathy

3. A 17-year-old male football player suddenly loses consciousness during a game. Cardiac workup reveals the patient has hypertrophic obstructive cardiomyopathy (HOCM).

Question 3a

Do you expect this patient to have a normal ejection fraction (EF)?

Answer 3a

No, most patients with HOCM have an elevated EF of ~80% due to the hypercontractile state of the heart.

Question 3b

What cardiac abnormalities are present in a patient with HOCM?

Answer 3b

Usually, patients with HOCM have dynamic left ventricular outflow obstruction (due to a hypertrophied myocardium), mitral regurgitation (due to systolic anterior movement of the mitral valve), diastolic dysfunction, myocardial ischemia, and dysrhythmias.

Coarctation of the Aorta

4. A 32-year-old G1P0 presents to you in the labor and delivery suite for induction of labor. Her past medical history includes coarctation of the aorta.

Question 4a

Would you use a regional anesthetic in this patient?

Answer 4a

Yes, I would. General or regional anesthesia is possible in a patient with coarctation of the aorta as long as abrupt hemodynamic changes do not occur, which can contribute to aortic dissection.

Question 4b

You decide on a regional technique for the case. Would you administer a spinal or an epidural?

Answer 4b

I would perform an epidural technique as it would allow me to slowly titrate dilute local anesthetic and prevent the abrupt sympathectomy associated with a spinal. Patients with coarctation of the aorta often have a lower pressure distal to the coarctation than proximal, so I would be wary of lowering her blood pressure suddenly.

Intra-Aortic Balloon Pump (IABP)

5. A 72-year-old female has an intra-aortic balloon pump (IABP) placed after a long, four-vessel on-pump CABG procedure.

Question 5a

Please describe how an IABP works.

Answer 5a

An IABP is a counterpulsation device that sits in the aorta and works by deflating during systole, thereby reducing afterload, and inflates in diastole, thereby increasing perfusion to the coronary arteries. The net result of these actions is that there is a decrease in myocardial work and an improvement in oxygen supply to the myocardium.

Question 5b

What are the contraindications to an IABP?

Answer 5b

Contraindications to an IABP can be divided into relative and absolute. The absolute contraindications are severe aortic valve insufficiency, aortic dissection, and aortoiliac disease. Relative contraindications are prosthetic vascular grafts in the aorta and vascular aneurysms at the site of insertion.

Automatic Implantable Cardioverter-Defibrillator (AICD)

6. A 66-year-old male presents for a laparoscopic cholecystectomy. He has an AICD in place.

Question 6a

How would you evaluate this patient's AICD preoperatively?

Answer 6a

I would perform a focused history and physical. I want to know his baseline cardiovascular status and the indication for the AICD. I would also want to know how often it has fired and when it was last interrogated. I would also look to see if this is just an AICD or if there is a pacemaker component. I would also contact the manufacturer to see if there are any special precautions I need to take, beyond what is routine for an AICD, that are specific to this device in the patient.

Question 6b

How does the presence of an AICD affect your intraoperative management?

Answer 6b

This patient is having surgery in the upper abdomen, which may come within 6 inches of the device. Depending on the AICD model, I would want to place a magnet over the AICD to inactivate it and have defibrillation pads on the patient in the event that he needs to be shocked. I would ask the surgeon to avoid electrocautery when possible and, if absolutely needed, to use short bursts. I would also ask for a bipolar electrocautery and communicate frequently with the surgeon to place the magnet only when electrocautery is about to occur, to minimize the amount of time that the AICD is disabled.

Cardiopulmonary Bypass (CPB)

7. A 65-year-old male is scheduled to undergo a four-vessel CABG. He has a history of diabetes, cholesterol, and hypertension.

Question 7a

Briefly describe the cardiopulmonary bypass machine.

Answer 7a

The CPB machine consists of a venous reservoir where deoxygenated blood collects from the patient via a venous cannula and is then transferred to an oxygenator where it is oxygenated. The oxygenated blood is then pumped through a main pump into an arterial filter. From the arterial filter, blood is pumped through an arterial cannula back into the patient.

Question 7b

Which type of oxygenator would you choose if you had the option for your bypass machine, a membrane or a bubble?

Answer 7b

If I had the option, I would choose a membrane oxygenator over a bubble oxygenator because in a membrane oxygenator gas is exchanged through a semipermeable silicon membrane and is therefore less traumatic to the blood. In a bubble oxygenator, small oxygen bubbles are formed and more trauma is endured by the red blood cells.

Abdominal Aortic Aneurysm (AAA)

8. A 55-year-old patient presents for open repair of an abdominal aortic aneurysm.

Question 8a

What steps can be taken to protect the patient's spinal cord during aortic cross-clamp?

Answer 8a

To protect the spinal cord, I would (1) monitor and maintain adequate BP above and below the cross-clamp; (2) institute hypothermia; (3) use CSF drainage to optimize spinal cord perfusion pressure (SCPP), which is defined as Aortic Pressure (AP) – Cerebrospinal Fluid (CSF) or Cerebral Venous Pressure (CVP) (whichever is greater); (4) request the surgeon to place a shunt across the cross-clamp to improve perfusion distal to the clamp; and (5) avoid vasodilators and inhalation agents that can increase intracranial pressure (ICP) and, thereby, spinal cord perfusion pressure (SCPP).

Question 8b

Would you place an epidural for this case? What are your concerns?

Answer 8b

Assuming the patient has no contraindications to a neuraxial technique such as anticoagulant therapy, back surgery, or absolute refusal of technique, I would place one. The benefits of placing one is that it allows for better post-operative pain control, improved respiratory function and pulmonary toilet postoperatively, decreased incidence of DVT, and improved GI function. However, it can also lead to hypotension secondary to a sympathectomy, so I would be cautious in administering local anesthesia perioperatively. I would also be cognizant of the fact that this patient may develop a coagulopathy postoperatively, preventing me from removing an epidural catheter as quickly as I would like.

Down Syndrome

9. A 42-year-old male with Down syndrome presents for an emergency appendectomy.

Question 9a

What are the cardiac considerations in patients with Down syndrome?

Answer 9a

Patients with Down syndrome are at an increased risk of endocardial cushion defects, ASD, VSD, PDA, or tetralogy of Fallot. Uncorrected defects can lead to pulmonary hypertension and Eisenmenger's complex.

Question 9b

Why are these patients at risk for pulmonary hypertension?

Answer 9b

These patients are at risk for pulmonary hypertension because they are at risk of having a congenital left-to-right shunt, which causes an increase in right-sided pressures to compensate for the shunted blood. Over time, this causes an increase in pulmonary artery pressures, progressing to pulmonary hypertension.

Bacterial Endocarditis

10. A 21-year-old female presents for a dilation and curettage. She has a history of mitral valve prolapse.

Question 10a

Does this patient need bacterial endocarditis prophylaxis?

Answer 10a

No. This patient is undergoing a genitourinary (GU) procedure, and administration of antibiotics solely to prevent infective endocarditis is no longer recommended for GU procedures.

Question 10b

What are the indications for bacterial endocarditis prophylaxis?

Answer 10b

Indications for endocarditis prophylaxis are patients with certain cardiac conditions who are undergoing certain procedures involving skin or mucosa (dental, skin, respiratory mucosa). The cardiac conditions are patients with a prosthetic valve or prosthetic material used for repair of a valve, previous endocarditis, congenital heart disease, unrepaired cyanotic disease, completely repaired congenital heart defect with prosthetic material during the first 6 months after the procedure, repaired congenital heart defect with residual defect, and cardiac transplant patients who develop a valvulopathy.

Suggested References

Atchabahian A, Gupta R, eds. *The Anesthesia Guide*. New York: McGraw Hill; 2013.

Barash PG, Cullen BF, Stoelting RK, Cahalan M, Stock CM. eds. *Clinical Anesthesia*. 6th ed. Philadelphia, PA: Lippincott Williams & Wilkins; 2009.

Hines RL, Marschall KE. eds. *Stoelting's Anesthesia and Coexisting Disease*. 5th ed. Philadelphia, PA: Elsevier; 2008.

34 Additional Topics: Obstetrics

Anita Gupta and Nicholas Weber

Cystic Fibrosis

1. A 22-year-old G1P0 female presents to the labor and delivery ward for induction. She has had no prenatal care throughout the 34 weeks of gestation. Her past medical history is significant for cystic fibrosis (CF). The pregnancy has been uncomplicated and the patient is currently resting comfortably in bed.

Question 1a

What are some important preoperative lab values to obtain for the CF patient?

Answer 1a

I would want coagulation studies and serum glucose levels because CF patients often have poor hepatic function and are unable to absorb fat-soluble vitamins, for example, vitamin K. Either of these issues may lead to coagulopathy. Many patients will be supplemented with the fat-soluble vitamins (A, D, E, K) during their pregnancy. Gestational diabetes is also common due to poor exocrine function. Oral glucose tolerance tests should be performed in each trimester, up until 30 weeks' gestation.

Question 1b

What complications may arise in a newborn with CF?

Answer 1b

Intestinal obstruction may be the first presenting sign of CF in a newborn. Thickened meconium can accrue in utero, which may obstruct the mid ileum. This leads to proximal dilation and bowel wall thickening. Complications such as volvulus, atresia, necrosis, perforation, meconium peritonitis, and pseudocyst formation may result.

Multiple Sclerosis

2. A 34-year-old G3P2 female presents to labor and delivery for premature uterine contractions. She is 31 weeks pregnant and her prenatal care has been complete and unremarkable. She has a history of multiple sclerosis (MS) for the past 9 years, and has been ambulating with a cane for the last 4 years.

Question 2a

How does pregnancy alter the disease state?

Answer 2a

Incidence of MS relapse decreases during pregnancy, most pronounced in the third trimester, and then may increase in the first 3 months postpartum.

Question 2b

What are the considerations when choosing an anesthetic for the parturient?

Answer 2b

MS has implications for both regional and general anesthesia. For regional, an epidural anesthetic can be placed, but a spinal anesthetic should be avoided because of the possibility of disease exacerbation. Regarding general anesthesia, I would be hesitant to administer a depolarizing muscle relaxant because of the potential for an exaggerated release of potassium. I would instead administer an NDMR with close attention to her twitches. For either technique, I would be careful to avoid infection and fever as these are associated with an exacerbation of MS.

Epilepsy

3. A 26-year-old G1P0 female at 39 weeks' gestation presents to labor and delivery in active labor. Her exam reveals that she is 2 cm dilated, +1, thick, and high. She has a history of epilepsy but has not been taking her medications because she has been nervous about the side effects to her child.

Question 3a

If the mother experiences a seizure at this moment, would you treat it with propofol?

Answer 3a

No. Propofol has a high apnea potential, which is not ideal in a pregnancy state because of an anticipated difficult airway. Instead, I would administer midazolam to treat the seizures.

Question 3b

What are the possible fetal repercussions of maternal epilepsy?

Answer 3b

The repercussion of maternal epilepsy is that the incidence of congenital malformations, such as fetal hydantoin syndrome, is about two and a half times more in neonates born to epileptic mothers. The syndrome includes intrauterine growth restriction (IUGR), skull and facial abnormalities, potential cleft lip/palate, and hypoplasia of nails and digits. Also, epileptic seizures can result in fetal asphyxia depending on their severity and progression to status epilepticus, which may have a maternal mortality of 10–25%.

Pre-eclampsia

4. A 41-year-old female G1P0 who is 35 weeks pregnant has been referred to labor and delivery for induction by her obstetrician. Her blood pressure in the outpatient office was 162/102 mmHg. Also, her urine dipstick was positive for +2 protein.

Question 4a

Explain the spectrum of syndromes described by pregnancy-induced hypertension (PIH).

Answer 4a

PIH describes three syndromes: pre-eclampsia, eclampsia, and HELLP.

Pre-eclampsia is defined by a triad that occurs after the 20th week of gestation. The first is sustained systolic blood pressure greater than 140/90 mmHg for mild pre-eclampsia and greater than 160/110 mmHg for severe pre-eclampsia. The second is proteinuria >2 g/day for mild, and >5 g/day for severe pre-eclampsia. The last part of the triad is generalized edema.

Eclampsia is defined as hypertension complicated by grand mal seizures.

HELLP is a syndrome described by hypertension with hemolysis, elevated liver enzymes, and low platelets.

Question 4b

What is the treatment for acute-onset severe hypertension with pre-eclampsia?

Answer 4b

As with any patient, the other vital signs must be assessed to ensure the patient is not hypoxic, hypercarbic, or in a malignant arrhythmia. If the patient is in pain, regional or IV pain medicines should be given. If the patient was anxious, I would provide verbal reassurance. If all of these potential causes were negative, I would conclude that the likely cause of the patient's hypertension is PIH. The treatment for that would be labetalol and hydralazine.

Anticoagulation in the Parturient

5. A 24-year-old female presents to the labor ward from the emergency department after her "water broke." She is 39 weeks and 2 days pregnant. She has a history of DVT and is on anticoagulation therapy.

Question 5a

What guidelines would you use to determine if neuraxial anesthesia is acceptable?

Answer 5a

It depends on her anticoagulant regiment. Low-molecular-weight heparin (LMWH) should be held for 12 hours prior to neuraxial procedures, and held for 12 hours before catheter removal. If high-dose LMWH is used: enoxaparin 1 mg/kg q12 hours or 1.5 mg/kg q day, dalteparin 120 U/kg q 12 hours, dalteparin 200 U/kg, or tinzaparin 175 U/kg, then dosing should be held for 24 hours. For thienopyridine therapy, ticlopidine should be held for 14 days and clopidogrel for 7 days. ASA and NSAIDs alone appear to give no added risk. Coumadin is contraindicated during pregnancy because of its category X designation by the US Food and Drug Administration (FDA).

Question 5b

What are the additional risks of general versus neuraxial anesthesia?

Answer 5b

General anesthesia has a mortality rate that is 16 times higher than that with neuraxial anesthesia. The major sources of mortality are attributed to hypoxia from failure to intubate the trachea and aspiration pneumonia. Additional risk factors for general anesthesia in the pregnant patient include asthma, upper respiratory tract infection, obesity, and history of difficult intubation. Apgar scores at 1 minute are lower after general anesthesia; however, no decrement in 5-minute Apgar scores has been shown.

Surgery in the Pregnant Patient

6. A 28-year-old female who is 26 weeks pregnant presents to the emergency department with acute cholecystitis. Prenatal care has shown no fetal issues during the pregnancy. Fetal heart rate monitoring indicates no current fetal distress. The patient is in moderate distress and has been NPO for more than 8 hours.

Question 6a

Surgery during which trimester carries the most risks?

Answer 6a

Surgery during the first trimester carries the most risk because this is when organogenesis occurs. In addition, the first trimester carries the highest risk for spontaneous abortions.

Question 6b

Do you still need to perform a rapid sequence induction (RSI) on this patient knowing that she has been NPO for more than 8 hours?

Answer 6b

Yes. I would still perform an RSI on this patient. There are several factors that decrease the GI transit time for this pregnant woman: gravid uterus, sympathetic nervous system greater than parasympathetic nervous system from the painful cholecystitis, and narcotics given to the patient in the ER to treat the pain.

Labor Epidural

7. A 23-year-old G1P0 female requests a labor epidural for vaginal delivery. The obstetricians tell you that the patient has been compliant with all of her prenatal care, and she has had no obstetric issues. While completing your history and physical she denied any past medical or surgical history.

Question 7a

What are the absolute and relative contraindications to epidural analgesia?

Answer 7a

Absolute: Patient refusal, sepsis with hemodynamic instability, uncorrected hypovolemia with ongoing hemorrhage, coagulopathy

Relative: Elevated intracranial pressure, prior back injury with neurological deficit, progressive neurological disease, for example, multiple sclerosis, chronic back pain, localized infection at the injection site

Question 7b

What physiological changes are expected with an epidural anesthesia?

Answer 7b

The physiological changes that are expected are as follows: (1) sympathectomy can result in reduced afterload and a decrease in blood pressure, with possible reflex tachycardia; (2) vasodilation may also decrease core temperature, leading to shivering; (3) unopposed parasympathetics may cause bladder distention and contraction of the bowel; and (4) decreased awareness of the motions of breathing may lead to the feeling of dyspnea.

Uterine Atony

8. A 35-year-old female G6P5 is currently undergoing a cesarean section for failure to progress. The patient is being managed in the operating room with a working epidural and she appears comfortable. A healthy baby was delivered. Immediately after removal of the placenta you estimate the blood loss to be greater than 1000 mL.

Question 8a

What are the risk factors for uterine atony?

Answer 8a

Uterine atony is failure of the uterus to contract after delivery. Atony is associated with overdistention of the uterus. Thus, the risk factors for uterine atony are multiparity, polyhydramnios, chorioamnionitis, augmented labor, large infants, and retained placenta.

Question 8b

How is uterine atony managed?

Answer 8b

Initially, bimanual compression and uterine massage is performed by the obstetric team. Pharmacologically, oxytocin is the first line, then intramuscular methylergonovine. For refractory uterine atony 15-methylprostaglandin F2-alpha may be given intramyometrially or intramuscularly. Coagulation factors may need replacement. Uterine bleed refractory to pharmacological measures is then controlled by ligation of the hypogastric arteries. The final measure is hysterectomy.

Aortic Stenosis

9. A 24-year-old full-term female with congenital aortic stenosis is requesting an epidural for labor analgesia. Pelvic ultrasound has revealed IUGR. The patient has not received prenatal care, and she is uncomfortable from her contractions.

Question 9a

What are the normal hemodynamic changes of pregnancy?

Answer 9a

The hemodynamic changes of pregnancy are associated with an increase in intravascular fluid volume. Anemia of pregnancy is a consequence of plasma volume increasing by 45% and erythrocyte volume increasing by 20%. Cardiac output increases by 50% by the third trimester and by 80% postpartum. Stroke volume is increased by 30% and heart rate is increased by 15–25%. Systemic vascular resistance decreases by 15%. As a consequence of these shifts, mean arterial blood pressure (MAP) may decrease by 15 mmHg, largely owing to a decrease in diastolic blood pressure.

Question 9b

Describe the hemodynamics of fixed aortic outflow obstruction and the theoretical issues that are complicated by neuraxial anesthesia.

Answer 9b

Coronary perfusion pressure (CPP) is defined as aortic diastolic blood pressure (aortDBP) – left ventricular end diastolic pressure (LVEDP). In aortic stenosis, the LVEDP is elevated, causing a decrease in CPP. Thus, to maintain CPP it is important to maintain the aortic BP, which correlates to MAP. The complication with neuraxial anesthesia is that it results in vasodilation and a decrease in MAP. Thus, to maintain CPP, one must prehydrate the patient and have pressors on standby to correct any sudden drops in BP.

von Willebrand's Disease (vWD)

10. A 31-year-old female who is 37 weeks pregnant presents to labor and delivery with blood seeping through her pants. She professes that she has von Willebrand disease. Previous hemoglobin levels have been in the normal range.

Question 10a

Describe Von Willebrand disease.

Answer 10a

Von Willebrand disease is a qualitative and/or quantitative defect in Von Willebrand factor (vWF), which stabilizes factor VIII, thereby promoting clotting. Type 1 is the most common type and is believed to be due to a decrease in actual vWF. Most patients with this type are asymptomatic. Type 2 is due to a qualitative defect in vWF and again is not clinically significant. Type 3 is the most severe form and is due to a virtual absence of vWF, resulting in mucosal hemorrhage, hemarthrosis, and hematomas.

Question 10b

What can be used to attenuate the bleeding in this patient?

Answer 10b

Depending on the type of von Willibrand disease, different treatment modalities are available. For type 1, pregnancy itself will increase circulating levels of vWF. Also, DDAVP is used to stimulate release of vWF from endothelial cells and is helpful with type 1 patients. For types 2 and 3 or if the patient is a nonresponder to DDAVP, cryoprecipitate, FFP, or factor VIII–vWF concentrates (Humate P) may be used.

Suggested Readings

Barash P, Cullen B, Stoelting R. *Clinical Anesthesia*. 5th ed. Philadelphia: Lippincott Williams & Wilkins; 2006.

Devonshire V, Duquette P, Dwosh E, Guimond C, Sadovnik AD. The immune system and hormones: review and relevance to pregnancy and contraception in women with MS. *Int Mult Scler J*. 2003;10:61–66.

Donaldson JO. Neurologic emergencies in pregnancy. *Obstet Gynecol*. 1997;177:1–7.

Duke J. *Anesthesia Secrets*. 3rd ed. St. Louis, MO: Mosby Elsevier; 2006.

Edenborough FP, Stableforth DE, Webb AK, et al. Outcome of pregnancy in women with cystic fibrosis. *Thorax*. 1995;50:170–174.

Goss CH, Rubenfeld GD, Otto K, et al. The effect of pregnancy on survival in women with cystic fibrosis. Chest. 2003;124: 1460–1468..

Hughes S, Levinson G, Rosen M. *Shinder and Levinson's Anesthesia for Obstetrics*. 4th ed. Philadelphia: Lippincott Williams & Wilkins; 2002.

Irish M, Reynolds M. Surgical aspects of cystic fibrosis and meconium ileus. Medscape 2015. https://emedicine.medscape.com/article/939603-overview.

Mygind KI, Mogens D, Christiansen J. Phenytoin and phenobarbitone plasma clearance during pregnancy. *Acta Neurol Scand.* 1976;54:160–166.

Reed A, Yudkowitz F. *Clinical Cases in Anesthesia.* 3rd ed. St. Louis, MO: Elsevier Churchill Livingstone; 2005.

Stoelting R, Dierdorf S. *Anesthesia and Co-Existing Diseases.* 4th ed. St. Louis, MO: Elsevier Churchill Livingstone; 2002.

Stoelting R, Miller R. *Basics of Anesthesia.* 5th ed. St. Louis, MO: Churchill Livingstone Elsevier; 2007.

Verma A, Das M, Ahluwalia A, et al. Pregnancy and cystic fibrosis. Cystic Fibrosis Trust. 2004. cfmedicine.com/htmldocs/CFText/pregnancy.htm.

35 Additional Topics: Pediatrics

Ruchir Gupta, Monique Cadogan, and Barbara Vickers

Malignant Hyperthermia

1. A 5-year-old boy presents to your ambulatory surgery center for a tonsillectomy and adenoidectomy. His father tells you that the patient's mother died of a "fever" during surgery.

Question 1a

Would you delay the case to perform a muscle biopsy on the child?

Answer 1a

No. Based on the information given, I would treat this child as malignant hyperthermia (MH) susceptible and avoid all triggering agents. Thus, a muscle biopsy would not change my management. In addition, the cost and discomfort associated with the biopsy may not be tolerated by the patient and family. This surgery can be safely executed with nontriggering agents and a muscle biopsy is not needed.

Question 1b

Would you insist this case be performed at a pediatric hospital instead of an ambulatory surgical center?

Answer 1b

No. This surgery can be safely conducted in an ambulatory surgical center provided that the necessary precautions are taken: avoidance of triggering agents, availability of an MH cart, and availability of supportive, resuscitative, and monitoring equipment.

2. An 8-year-old female with a history of King-Denborough syndrome presents for an emergency appendectomy. She has never had surgery before.

Question 2a

What are the principle anesthetic considerations in this patient?

Answer 2a

The principle anesthetic consideration in this patient is that she is susceptible to MH because of her history of King-Denborough syndrome. Thus, all triggering agents should be avoided and the MH cart should be readily available.

Question 2b

What steps will you take to reduce the chance of this patient developing malignant hyperthermia?

Answer 2b

There are several things that I would do to reduce the risk. First, I would remove all triggering agents such as succinycholine and volatile anesthetic vaporizers from the room. I would also flush out my anesthesia machine with 100% O_2 to remove any residual gases. Next, I would review the contents of the MH cart, making sure the drugs are all up to date and have not expired. Then, I would have a team meeting with the nurses, surgeons, and any residents/fellows to delegate roles if an MH episode did occur. Finally, I would inform the PACU that an MH-susceptible patient is about to have surgery and they should reserve a bed in the ICU in the event an emergent transfer is needed. If I am working in a hospital that does not have a pediatric ICU, I would also contact the nearest tertiary care center and request to have a bed available in case the patient needs to be emergently transferred.

CHARGE Syndrome

3. A 5-year-old Mexican male is scheduled for a cochlear implant. The child was brought to the United States by a religious mission that is funding his care. He has a history of CHARGE syndrome.

Question 3a

What are the airway considerations for a patient with CHARGE syndrome?

Answer 3a

Patients with CHARGE syndrome commonly have a cleft lip and palate. In addition, they may also present with micrognathia, laryngomalacia, subglottic stenosis, recurrent laryngeal nerve palsy, tracheomalacia, and tracheoesophageal fistula. Care must be taken to identify which of these abnormalities are present. The difficult-airway equipment should be on standby along with an ENT surgeon for an emergent tracheostomy.

Question 3b

Will you insist on an echocardiogram before taking this patient to the OR?

Answer 3b

Yes, I would want an echocardiogram in this patient because up to 75% of patients with CHARGE syndrome have concomitant cardiac defects. These defects can be simple but can also be very complex, such as tetralogy of Fallot.

Treacher-Collins Syndrome

4. A 4-year-old patient with a history of Treacher-Collins syndrome presents for an emergency appendectomy.

Question 4a

What are the major differences between the Treacher-Collins and Pierre-Robin syndromes?

Answer 4a

Both syndromes are associated with micrognathia and difficult airways, but Pierre-Robin syndrome is also known for glossoptosis. In addition, while cardiac defects occur with increased frequency in both populations, other congenital defects are more common with Treacher-Collins syndrome than with Pierre-Robin syndrome.

Question 4b

How are you going to secure the airway in this patient?

Answer 4b

These patients are known to have difficult airways. Thus, I would have the difficult-airway cart in the room, with the neck prepped and draped with a tracheostomy kit open and ready. Then, I would administer PO midazolam and perform a sedated fiber-optic intubation while maintaining spontaneous ventilations. If the patient remained uncooperative, I would administer titrating doses of ketamine and glycopyrrolate while maintaining spontaneous ventilations. Once the patient was sedated, I would use my fiber-optic scope to visualize the vocal cords and insert the ETT.

Tetralogy of Fallot

5. A 3-year-old male patient is scheduled for a cardiac catheterization. The patient's mother states that the child frequently "turns blue."

Question 5a

What may explain this finding?

Answer 5a

When venous blood bypasses the lungs and returns to the systemic circulation (right-to-left shunting) patients are at risk of cyanosis.

Question 5b

How does a right-to-left cardiac shunt impact intravenous induction? Inhalational induction?

Answer 5b

A patient with a right-to-left shunt would have a faster intravenous induction and a slower inhalation induction. To reduce further intraoperative right-to-left intracardiac shunting, higher systemic vascular resistance is utilized.

Pyloric Stenosis

6. A 3-week-old female with pyloric stenosis requires a laparoscopic pyloromyotomy. She is full term and otherwise healthy.

Question 6a

What would you expect her chemistry panel to show?

Answer 6a

I would expect a hypochloremic, hypokalemic, metabolic alkalosis secondary to persistent vomiting. In extreme cases where the dehydration is severe, this may progress to a metabolic acidemia secondary to hypoperfusion.

Question 6b

Assuming the patient is medically optimized, how would you induce this patient?

Answer 6b

Given the severe risk for aspiration, the stomach needs to be decompressed either via NG or OG tube in the lateral, supine, and prone positions to remove as much of the gastric contents as possible. After preoxygenating the child with 100% O_2 and atropine to prevent a vagal response to direct laryngoscopy, I would perform a rapid sequence induction with propofol and rocuronium.

Airway Management

7. You are paged by the PACU nurse for a 4-year-old female status post tonsillectomy and adenoidectomy who has been vomiting blood. Her BP is 63/32 mmHg while supine, heart rate 134 bpm, and respiratory rate 24.

Question 7a

Once the child is brought back to the OR, how would you induce this patient?

Answer 7a

For induction, I would choose agents that provide the best hemodynamic support given this patient's unstable vital signs and full-stomach status. After preoxygenating with 100% O_2, I would perform a rapid sequence intubation with cricoid pressure using ketamine and rocuronium.

Question 7b

Your resident suggests using succinycholine because this patient's airway needs to be rapidly secured because of her bleeding tonsil. How do you respond?

Answer 7b

I would inform the resident that while the airway is concerning, rocuronium in adequate doses can provide similar paralytic onset time to that of succinycholine. Succinycholine carries the additional risk of precipitating malignant hyperthermia in this patient if there is an undiagnosed myopathy. Thus, the risks of succinycholine outweigh the benefits.

Down Syndrome–Preoperative Evaluation

8. A 2-year-old male with Down syndrome presents for a left inguinal hernia repair.

Question 8a

What are your preoperative concerns in this patient?

Answer 8a

Down syndrome has clinical manifestations in just about every major organ system. My concerns are as follows:

Airway: These patients often have macroglossia and subglottic stenosis, both of which contribute to a potentially difficult airway.

GI: If this patient has duodenal atresia, I would treat him as having a full stomach.

Cardiac: These patients often have coexisting endocardial cushion defects. I would want to know what coexisting cardiac defects he has since this will affect my choice of induction/maintenance agents. A baseline echocardiogram might be warranted.

Neurological: These patients can have atlantoaxial subluxation. Thus, I would want to maintain this patient's neck in the neutral position and avoid any maneuvers that can strain or place pressure on the neck.

Respiratory: Obstructive airway disease is often present in these patients and they are more prone to snoring and apnea. These patients are also at increased risk for infection, vision loss, and hearing loss.

Question 8b

During the neurological evaluation, you notice the patient has a positive Babinski sign. Does this concern you?

Answer 8b

Yes, it does. A positive Babinski sign argues strongly for the possibility of neurological compromise in this patient, most likely secondary to the atlantoaxial subluxation. I would inform the parents that such a condition increases this patient's risk for perioperative neurological compromise. It would be wise to reschedule this elective case once the patient has been evaluated by a neurologist.

Down Syndrome—Intraoperative Management

9. A 4-year-old patient with Down syndrome presents for a tonsillectomy and adenoidectomy.

Question 9a

How would you secure the airway in this patient?

Answer 9a

Before the patient is brought into the OR, I would make sure the emergency airway cart is in the room as well as the ENT surgeon. After a careful airway exam, I would perform an inhalational induction with oxygen and sevoflurane. Once the child is mask induced and an IV established, I would keep the neck neutral and avoid neck extension during the direct laryngoscopy.

Question 9b

The patient had a tetralogy of Fallot repaired at 2 years of age. Does this patient need infective endocarditis (IE) prophylaxis?

Answer 9b

No. IE prophylaxis is only indicated in patients with certain cardiac conditions who are undergoing dental procedures. IE prophylaxis is warranted in patients with a history of prosthetic valve or prosthetic material used for repair of a valve, previous endocarditis, congenital heart disease (unrepaired cyanotic disease), completely repaired congenital heart defect with prosthetic material during first 6 months after procedure, repaired congenital heart defect with residual defect, and cardiac transplant patients who develop a valvulopathy.

Omphalocele

10. A 5 kg, 1-day-old male presents for closure of an omphalocele.

Question 10a

What are the key difference between an omphalocele and a gastroschisis?

Answer 10a

There are several differences between an omphalocele and a gastroschisis. First, an omphalocele is usually located within the umbilical cord, whereas a gastroschisis is to the right of it. Second, an omphalocele has a membranous sac covering it, whereas in gastroschisis there is no covering and the viscera is exposed. Finally, an omphalocele is associated with several conditions, including Beckwith-Wiedemann syndrome, congenital heart disease, trisomy 13, 18, and 21, and Pentalogy of Cantrell. Gastroschisis, by contrast, is associated mainly with prematurity and intestinal atresia.

Question 10b

At the end of the procedure, the patient begins to desaturate as the abdomen is being closed. How will you respond?

Answer 10b

Based on the information given, it seems likely that the patient is desaturating owing to impaired pulmonary compliance from increased abdominal pressure from the wound closure. Thus, after making sure the other vitals were stable, I would immediately ask the surgeon to open the wound and relieve the abdominal pressure. A staged closure where only superficial layers are initially closed would then have to occur.

PEDIATRICS

Suggested Readings

American Society of Anesthesiologists. Practice advisory for the perioperative management of patients with cardiac implantable electronic devices: pacemakers and implantable cardioverter-defibrillators. An updated report by the American Society of Anesthesiologists Task Force on Perioperative Management of Patients with Cardiac Implantable Electronic Devices. *Anesthesiology*. 2011; 114: 247–261.

Barash PG, Cullen BF, Stoelting RK, Cahalan M, Stock CM, eds. *Clinical Anesthesia*. 6th ed. Philadelphia, PA: Lippincott Williams & Wilkins; 2009

Hines RL, Marschall KE, eds. *Stoelting's Anesthesia and Coexisting Disease*. 5th ed. Philadelphia, PA: Elsevier; 2008.

Touloukian RJ, Higgins E. The spectrum of serum electrolytes in hypertrophic pyloric stenosis. *J Pediatric Surg*. 1983;18(4):394–397.

36 Additional Topics: Neuroanesthesia

Ruchir Gupta

Cerebral Aneurysm

1. A 55-year-old male with a history of coronary artery disease (CAD) presents for emergency clipping of a partially ruptured cerebral aneurysm. On physical exam, he has a Mallampati 4 airway and limited neck movement secondary to a previous cervical fusion.

Question 1a

The surgeon asks you to perform a slow, controlled induction to avoid life-threatening hypertension (HTN) in this patient, which could cause aneurysmal rupture. How do you respond?

Answer 1a

I would inform the surgeon that this patient is not a candidate for a slow, controlled induction because of his difficult airway. I would also tell the surgeon that to ensure the patient has stable hemodynamics during the awake intubation, I will perform airway blocks (superior laryngeal/recurrent laryngeal), administer nebulized lidocaine, and have a preinduction A-line with an esmolol drip attached to emergently treat any rise in BP during the intubation.

Question 1b

During dissection of the aneurysm, the patient's BP is 100/60 mmHg. The surgeon asks you to lower the BP further to aid in the dissection. How do you respond?

Answer 1b

My concern in this patient is to maintain a BP that is sufficiently low to perfuse the coronary arteries without inducing myocardial ischemia. Thus, I will look at the current BP and corresponding EKG to rule out signs of myocardial ischemia. Then, I will begin to administer nitroglycerin or esmolol infusion slowly while looking at the EKG for any signs of ischemia. I would also ask the surgeon to place a temporary clip on the feeding vessel to lower the amount of blood entering the aneurysm.

Intracranial Tumor

2. A 67-year-old female presents for resection of an intracranial tumor.

Question 2a

What are the components of intracranial pressure (ICP)?

Answer 2a

ICP is composed of cerebral tissue, CSF, and cerebral blood volume.

Question 2b

How would you determine if this patient has an elevated ICP preoperatively?

Answer 2b

Preoperatively, I would perform a focused history and physical. In the history, I would ask the patient if she has had any nausea or vomiting, weakness in any part of her body, or any headaches. From the physical, I would want to know if there have been any changes in mentation from baseline. Any evidence of somnolence will strongly argue for an elevated ICP. I would also examine for the presence of papilledema and focal neurological deficits, such as nerve palsy or muscle weakness.

Autonomic Hyperreflexia

3. A surgeon wishes to perform an incision and drainage (I&D) of a chronic heel ulcer on a paraplegic patient with a T4 spinal cord transection.

Question 3a

The surgeon asks you to just administer 2 mg of midazolam, as the patient has no sensation below the level of the lesion. How do you respond?

Answer 3a

I would inform the surgeon that administering midazolam alone would not be sufficient anesthesia for this patient because this patient is at high risk for autonomic hyperreflexia. Autonomic hyperreflexia can only be prevented by removing the surgical stimulus or administering a deep general anesthetic so as to prevent the patient from feeling the surgical stimulus.

Question 3b

What is the pathogenesis of autonomic hyperreflexia?

Answer 3b

Autonomic hyperreflexia results from a stimulus below the level of transection causing sympathetically mediated HTN, bradycardia, sweating, and flushing above the lesion.

Cerebral Vasospasm

4. A 70-year-old male underwent aneurysm clipping for a subarachnoid hemorrhage 1 day ago and has been in the neurosurgical ICU overnight, intubated and sedated.

NEUROANESTHESIA

Question 4a

What are the major postoperative concerns you would have for this patient?

Answer 4a

These patients are at high risk for the development of seizures, so antiseizure prophylaxis is given. They are also at high risk for rebleeding, so BP must be controlled. Hydrocephalus is also a concern and is treated with ventricular drainage. Finally, vasospasm is common typically from days 3 to 15 post-bleed, and daily sonographic exams must be performed to detect vasospasm.

Question 4b

What is meant by the term *triple H therapy*?

Answer 4b

Triple H therapy refers to hypertension, hypervolemia, and hemodilution. This therapy is indicated as treatment for cerebral vasospasm.

TURP Syndrome

5. A 54-year-old male is undergoing a transurethral retrograde prostatectomy (TURP) under spinal anesthesia.

Question 5a

What steps can you take to minimize this patient's risk of developing TURP syndrome?

Answer 5a

To minimize the risk of TURP syndrome, I would make sure the height gradient between the irrigation fluid and the patient is minimized to reduce the hydrostatic procedure, limit the duration of the procedure, and maintain verbal contact with the patient throughout the procedure.

Question 5b

Midway through the case the patient becomes confused and tachycardic. You intubate and place an arterial line. A stat Na level comes back at 121 mEq/L. Will you administer hypertonic saline?

Answer 5b

No. Correction of Na must be gradual so as to prevent central pontine myelinolysis. At 121 mEq/L, I would begin with securing the airway, restricting fluid, administering Lasix, and evaluating for EKG changes. If the condition continued to deteriorate and his Na continued to decrease, I would consider administering hypertonic saline.

Pituitary Tumor

6. A 45-year-old male presents for resection of a growth hormone–secreting pituitary tumor.

Question 6a

What are your preoperative concerns regarding his condition?

Answer 6a

My concerns regarding his condition are that he may display signs of acromegaly, which would make it difficult to secure the airway. Also, this patient may have glottic stenosis, necessitating a smaller-diameter ETT, with proper tests for a leak to ensure there is no compression of the cuff on the tracheal mucosa. My non-airway concerns would be an increased incidence of CAD, HTN, obstructive sleep apnea (OSA), and insulin resistance in this patient. I would probe to see which of these conditions the patient has and how severe of an effect they have had on his organ systems so that I can tailor my anesthesia accordingly.

Question 6b

How will you secure the airway?

Answer 6b

Given this patient's risk for a difficult airway, I would want to perform an awake fiber-optic intubation in this patient. I would begin by administering 4% nebulized lidocaine, glycopyrrolate, and small, titrating doses of a benzodiazepine prior to placing the scope.

Electroconvulsive Therapy (ECT)

7. You are asked to provide anesthesia for a 39-year-old male with bipolar disorder. Upon reviewing this patient's medication list, you notice he has been on lithium.

Question 7a

Will you delay the case?

Answer 7a

Yes. Lithium must be withheld for 36–72 hours or else it may cause a prolongation of the seizure with resulting dysrhythmias or delirium.

Question 7b

On further questioning, the patient tells you that recently he has been urinating significantly more than he had in the past. Could this be related to his lithium?

Answer 7b

Yes. Lithium therapy is associated with diabetes insipidus. Treatment of lithium-induced diabetes insipidus is cessation or reduction of the offending agent.

Hyponatremia

8. A 34-year-old male underwent an open reduction of a right humerus after a severe motorcycle accident in which he wasn't wearing a helmet. A head CT scan reveals a small, stable subdural hematoma. On POD #2 his Na level is 127 mEq/L.

Question 8a

What is the mechanism of action of syndrome of inappropriate antidiuretic hormone (SIADH)?

Answer 8a

SIADH results from unregulated release of antidiuretic hormone (ADH), which acts on the distal convoluted tubule and the collecting duct to reabsorb water, not solute. The result is retention of water with a dilution of solute, leading to hyponatremia, decreased serum osmolarity, increased urine osmolarity, and decreased urine production.

Question 8b

How can you distinguish SIADH from cerebral salt wasting syndrome (CSWS)?

Answer 8b

Clinically, one would see hypovolemia in CSWS and euvolemia or hypervolemia in SIADH. In terms of lab studies, the urine osmolarity (UO) is high in SIADH and low to normal in CSWS. Furthermore, polyuria is seen in CSWS, whereas UO is decreased in SIADH.

Peripheral Neuropathy

9. A 47-year-old female complains of persistent left little finger weakness 1 week after her laparoscopic cholecystectomy.

Question 9a

How would you evaluate this patient?

Answer 9a

I would perform a focused history and physical. From the history, I would want to know when the symptoms began, whether they are getting better or worse, whether any pain accompanies the weakness, and whether there is also a sensory component. From the physical, I would examine the area for signs of infection or inflammation, assess muscle strength, and clearly delineate the area of the sensory loss with a marking pen.

Question 9b

Assuming this was an ulnar nerve injury secondary to malpositioning, how would you treat this?

Answer 9b

I would begin treatment with conservative measures as well as follow-up visits because most of these injuries are self-limiting. If the symptoms persisted or worsened, I would order EMG studies and request a neurology consult.

Multiple Sclerosis

10. A 38-year-old female with multiple sclerosis (MS) presents for a right hemicolectomy.

Question 10a

What precautions would you take to prevent exacerbation of her MS symptoms?

Answer 10a

To prevent exacerbation, I would avoid any increase in body temperature, whether iatrogenic or from an infection. I would exercise judicious use of antibiotics and ensure that the Bair hugger is not delivering too much warm air to the patient. I would also avoid using a spinal anesthetic in this patient because spinal techniques have been implicated in exacerbating symptoms. In the postoperative period, I would perform periodic neurological checks and ensure that the patient does not experience any rise in temperature.

Question 10b

Can this patient have neuraxial anesthesia for this case?

Answer 10b

Yes, this patient can have an epidural neuraxial block. For reasons that are unclear, patients with MS who receive spinal anesthesia experience an exacerbation of symptoms, whereas those with an epidural or peripheral nerve blocks do not. It is believed that this may be due to MS rendering the spinal cord more susceptible to the toxic effects of local anesthetics.

Suggested Readings

Atchabahian A, Gupta R. *The Anesthesia Guide*. New York: McGraw-Hill; 2013.

Cotrell JE, Young WL, eds. *Cottrell's Neuroanesthesia*. 5th ed. St. Louis, MO: Elsevier Health Sciences; 2010.

37 Additional Topics: Pain Management

Ruchir Gupta

Pain Onset

1. A 35-year-old female injured her shoulder during an ice skating accident. She presents today with persistent right arm pain.

Question 1a

What is the mechanism of peripheral nerve sensitization to pain? Central nervous sensitization?

Answer 1a

Tissue damage results in the release of inflammatory mediators, which sensitize peripheral nerves. Central sensitization refers to the increased synaptic efficacy in the spinal cord caused by intense painful stimuli or nerve damage. As a result, this increased synaptic transmission causes patients to have a lower threshold for pain, an increased sensation to otherwise mild pain, and increased sensitivity to pain in noninjured areas.

Question 1b

What is meant by allodynia?

Answer 1b

Allodynia is a pain sensation caused by a stimulus that does not normally provoke pain. This is different from hyperalgesia, an exaggerated reaction to a stimulus that is normally painful.

Chronic Pain

2. You are consulted on treating a 67-year-old patient with end-stage pancreatic cancer, now in hospice care. The primary care resident claims that multiple pain therapies have been attempted, but the patient continues to be in extreme pain all the time.

Question 2a

How would you evaluate this patient?

Answer 2a

I would perform a focused history and physical. From the history, I would want to know where the pain is located and its intensity, radiation, and coexisting symptoms. I would also want to know which medicines had been administered and what effect they have had on the pain. If the patient had any interventional pain management techniques, I would also want to know about that. From the physical, I would examine the patient to assess where exactly the pain is located. Although I am told this is from pancreatic cancer, I would also evaluate for other causes of the pain, such as inflammation from another cause at the site of the pain. Finally, I would look at imaging studies, such as a CT scan of the abdomen, to see if surgical debulking is a possibility.

Question 2b

Would you use opioids to treat this patient's pain?

Answer 2b

Yes. It appears that the patient is suffering from breakthrough pain despite multiple pain modalities (step 3 of the World Health Organization [WHO] pain ladder). I would administer opioids to acutely reduce her pain. Once her pain was under control, I would consult a pain specialist to develop a short- to intermediate-term pain plan for this patient.

Complex Regional Pain Syndrome (CRPS) Type 1

3. A patient is referred to your outpatient pain clinic for evaluation of a complex regional pain syndrome (CRPS).

Question 3a

What is complex regional pain syndrome?

Answer 3a

CRPS is a disease resulting from dysregulation of the cranial nerves, which leads to pain, burning, swelling, and changes in skin color and temperature. CRPS usually follows a relatively minor trauma, such as contusion, sprain, fracture, or dislocation.

Question 3b

How would you determine if this patient has CRPS 1 or 2?

Answer 3b

CRPS types 1 and 2 are distinguished mainly by the etiology. Whereas CRPS 1 can result from injury to any part of the body, CRPS type 2 results from injury to a nerve bundle. The pain onset is usually immediate and is associated with allodynia, hyperpathia, and vasomotor changes.

Stellate Ganglion

4. You are performing a stellate ganglion block on a 32-year-old female who developed CRPS in her right upper extremity.

Question 4a

Where is the stellate ganglion located?

Answer 4a

The stellate ganglion is located at the level of C7 (seventh cervical vertebrae), anterior to the transverse process of C7, anterior to the neck of the first rib, and just below the subclavian artery.

Question 4b

What are the possible complications associated with a stellate ganglion block?

Answer 4b

Complications of stellate ganglion blocks are intravascular injection, subarachnoid injection, hematoma, pneumothorax, brachial plexus block, hoarseness due to recurrent laryngeal nerve injury, and epidural block.

Myofascial Pain

5. A 48-year-old female has been receiving trigger point injections of steroid and local anesthetic in her upper back regions for myofacial pain.

Question 5a

What are trigger points?

Answer 5a

Trigger points are areas in the skeletal muscle that are hyperirritable. Often, palpable nodules in taut bands of muscle fibers are present with focal-point tenderness. Injection of local anesthetic at these points is the mainstay of treatment in patients with myofacial pain.

Question 5b

How does transcutaneous electrical nerve stimulation (TENS) therapy work?

Answer 5b

There are different proposed mechanisms for how TENS works. Inhibition of pain signals at presynaptic levels is one mechanism. Another mechanism involves electrical impulse stimulation, which causes the release of endogenous substances involved in pain control.

Opioids

6. A 36-year-old G1P0 female is on chronic methadone therapy. She is currently 36 weeks pregnant.

Question 6a

Should you stop her methadone to prevent neonatal narcotic dependency?

Answer 6a

No, I would not, because patients on chronic methadone therapy risk preterm labor, fetal distress, or fetal demise if abruptly discontinued. In fact, it has been suggested to increase the methadone dose during the third trimester because maternal volume of distribution is increased, leading to a dilutional effect of the methadone.

Question 6b

What are your concerns for her newborn?

Answer 6b

I am concerned that the newborn is at risk for neonatal abstinence syndrome (NAS). This syndrome manifests as increased sweating, nasal stuffiness, fever, temperature instability, tachypnea, mottling of the skin, tremors, irritability, increased wakefulness, high-pitched crying, myoclonus, hypertonicity and hyperactive reflexes, seizures, yawning, sneezing, and skin excoriation due to excessive rubbing. A small percentage may develop seizures. These patients may also have poor feeding, uncoordinated and constant sucking, vomiting or regurgitation, loose or watery stools, and dehydration.

Cancer Pain

7. A 72-year-old patient with end-stage pancreatic cancer presents for a celiac plexus block.

Question 7a

What are the side effects and complications of a celiac plexus block?

Answer 7a

Side effects and complications of a celiac plexus block include life-threatening hypotension secondary to the sympathectomy, hemorrhage from vascular injury, abdominal cramping and diarrhea from unopposed parasympathetic action, organ injury, local anesthetic toxicity, paraplegia from damage to the artery of Adamkiewicz, and neuronal injury.

Question 7b

If this patient had uterine cancer rather than pancreatic cancer, which block would you perform?

Answer 7b

In the case of uterine cancer, a superior hypogastric plexus block is used because the pain arises from the pelvic viscera.

Post-amputation Pain

8. A 26-year-old male is status posttraumatic left below-the-knee amputation, performed 6 weeks ago after a motor cycle accident. The patient continues to complain of pain in the left toes.

Question 8a

Your resident wants to call a psychiatry consult because the patient is complaining of pain in areas that no longer exist. Do you agree?

Answer 8a

No, I would not rush to call a psychiatry consult. This patient may be experiencing phantom limb pain, which is relatively common in post-amputee patients. Phantom limb pain is a complex syndrome with a wide array of sequelae ranging from severe pain to tingling and itching. Several theories have been advanced regarding the neurological basis, with no absolute consensus.

Question 8b

What is the treatment for phantom limb pain?

Answer 8b

There is no absolutely satisfactory treatment for this syndrome. Current treatment modalities include spinal cord stimulation, heat application, vibration therapy, acupuncture, physical therapy, hypnosis, biofeedback, and medications such as antidepressants, anticonvulsants, beta blockers, and sodium channel blockers.

Lower Back Pain and Sciatica

9. A 62-year-old construction worker presents to the interventional pain clinic with chronic lower back pain.

Question 9a

How would you evaluate the patient?

Answer 9a

I would perform a focused history and physical. From the history, I would want to know where the pain is, how severe it is on a scale of 1 to 10 and whether it is with or without radiation, any exacerbating or alleviating factors, and what treatment modalities he has attempted and their outcomes. From the physical, I would want to examine his back, looking for gross signs of inflammation (rubor, calor, dolor) as well as any gross deformities. I would also assess if the pain is tender to palpation.

Question 9b

An MRI ordered by his primary care physician shows an L5–S1 disc degeneration. He has been on NSAIDs, opioids, and physical therapy, with minimal relief. Recently, the pain has been radiating down his right leg. What treatment options would you offer this patient?

Answer 9b

I would review with him his past medications and assess if the maximum dose of opioids and nonopiod drugs had been met and if not, what side effects, if any, prevented the continued use of those drugs. In terms of procedures, I would discuss with the patient the possibility of a lumbar epidural steroid injection (LESI) to place medicine in the epidural space. If the symptoms were unilateral, a transformainal approach could be used.

Suggested Readings

Argoff CE, McCleane G, eds. *Pain Management Secrets*. 3rd ed. Philadelphia, PA: Mosby Elsevier; 2009.

Fishman SM, Ballantyne JC, Rathmell JP, eds. *Bonica's Management of Pain*. 4th ed. Philadelphia, PA: Lippincott Williams & Wilkins; 2009.

Miller RD, Eriksson LI, Fleisher LA, Wiener-Kornish JP, Young WL, eds. *Miller's Anesthesia*. 7th ed. Philadelphia, PA: Churchill Livingstone Elsevier; 2010.

Warfield CA, Bajwa ZH, eds. *Principles and Practice of Pain Medicine*. 2nd ed. New York: McGraw-Hill Medical Publishing Division; 2004.

38 Additional Topics: Neuraxial and Anticoagulation

Ruchir Gupta

Neuraxial in Patient with COPD

1. A 68-year-old patient with COPD and a 50 pack-year smoking history presents for a cystoscopy.

Question 1a

What is the best anesthetic technique for this patient?

Answer 1a

I would choose an epidural technique. The benefits of an epidural are avoidance of intubation and ventilatory support, fewer DVTs, better postoperative pain control, less systemic side effects from opioids, and quicker ambulation.

Question 1b

What information would you require before performing a neuraxial technique in this patient?

Answer 1b

I would want to know if this patient has any coagulopathies, is on any anticoagulant medication, has any history of nerve injuries, has had any back surgeries with or without instrumentation, and has had any problems with any neuraxial technique he underwent in the past.

Heparin with Patient-Controlled Epidural Analgesia (PCEA)

2. You are paged by a nurse of the medical floor to remove an epidural catheter in a patient with patient-controlled epidural analgesia (PCEA).

Question 2a

How long since the last heparin dose must you wait before removing the catheter?

Answer 2a

It depends on the type of heparin. If it is unfractionated subcutaneous heparin, there is no delay. If it is IV unfractionated heparin, then I would wait 2–4 hours. If it is LMWH low-dose QD dosing, then I would wait 12 hours. If it is low-dose BID dosing, I would have removed the catheter before initiating treatment. With LMWH at a high dose I would wait 24 hours.

Question 2b

How long will you require that the heparin for this patient be held after you remove the catheter?

Answer 2b

I would ask them to hold it for 1 hour if it is IV unfractionated heparin and 2 hours if it is LMWH, regardless of dose.

Neuraxial in Patient with CAD

3. A 55-year-old female with three cardiac stents presents for a right knee replacement. She is currently on Plavix and ASA for her CAD.

Question 3a

Which type of neuraxial technique would you use for this patient?

Answer 3a

I would not perform a neuraxial technique because such procedures are contraindicated in patients taking Plavix because of the risk of a neuraxial hematoma.

Question 3b

Would you perform a neuraxial technique on a patient taking just ASA?

Answer 3b

There is no contraindication to neuraxial technique in a patient using ASA.

Epidural in HELLP Syndrome

4. A G1P0 woman presents to the labor and delivery suite in labor. She was diagnosed recently with the HELLP syndrome.

Question 4a

Would you place an epidural in this patient?

Answer 4a

It depends. In addition to inquiring about the routine conditions that would preclude the use of an epidural, I would also want to perform a focused history and physical to ascertain the severity of her HELLP syndrome. From the history, I would want to know how long she has had this and if has she noticed any easy bruising or bleeding as a result. From the physical, I would look for signs of bruising. Finally, I would look at the lab results to see her platelet level and also a baseline coagulation profile.

Question 4b

What is your cutoff regarding the platelet number in this patient before performing a neuraxial technique?

Answer 4b

I do not have an absolute cutoff. Instead, I would want to trend the platelets if possible to see if they are stable or decreasing. I would also look for any signs and symptoms of thrombocytopenia.

Post-Dural Puncture Headache (PDHD)

5. You are paged by the obstetric team to evaluate a 23-year-old G1P1 woman with a post-dural puncture headache (PDHD).

Question 5a

What treatments are available for patients with PDHD?

Answer 5a

The only definitive treatment is a blood patch, but the majority of cases of PDHD resolve on their own if left untreated. Hydration, bed rest, caffeine, and Fioricet can all be given until the symptoms resolve on their own.

Question 5b

Describe how a blood patch is performed.

Answer 5b

A blood patch usually requires two clinicians: one to access the epidural space and the other to draw blood using sterile technique from the upper extremity. Communication between both clinicians is of paramount importance. The first clinician accesses the epidural space as if performing an epidural anesthetic. Once the space is accessed, the second clinician uses Betadine or an equivalent prepping solution to clean the area where the blood will be drawn. Using sterile gloves and equipment, 20 mL of blood is drawn into a syringe and handed to the first clinician, who then injects it through the epidural needle into the epidural space.

Neuraxial in Patient with CHF

6. A 75-year-old male with severe congestive heart failure (CHF) with an EF of 20% presents for a cystoscopy.

Question 6a

He wishes to remain awake and asks if he could have a spinal. How do you respond?

Answer 6a

I would not place a spinal in this patient because a spinal results in a sympathectomy, with venous pooling below the level of the spinal. As a result, there will be lower stroke volume for this patient, which will reduce his EF further and lead to cardiac compromise.

Question 6b

Could you place an epidural?

Answer 6b

An epidural would be a safer choice than a spinal because it allows me to slowly titrate in dilute concentrations of the anesthetic and assess the effect on the patient's cardiac status. Still, I would not want to risk compromising this patient's cardiac function further and would avoid all neuraxial techniques.

Thoracic Epidural

7. A 55-year-old female with small-cell carcinoma of the lung presents for a left lower lobectomy.

Question 7a

At what level would you place the epidural catheter for postoperative pain?

Answer 7a

Generally, the epidural is placed at the level of the incision or one to two levels lower.

Question 7b

Your resident asks you whether a spinal technique would be a better option. How do you respond?

Answer 7b

I would tell the resident that a spinal is not a better option than an epidural because an epidural allows for catheter placement, which will allow the titration of local anesthesia as well as narcotics during the case, thereby reducing the need for systemic anesthetics. It will also provide a conduit for administering postoperative pain. Additionally, a spinal anesthetic tends to be denser than an epidural and, at that level, could lead to difficulty in the use of muscles needed for adequate respiration and pulmonary toilet in the postoperative period.

Coumadin

8. You go to the ICU to remove an epidural catheter you placed 2 days earlier in a patient for postoperative pain. Upon arrival, you

learn that the surgical resident accidentally restarted this patient's Coumadin dose.

Question 8a

How does warfarin (Coumadin) work?

Answer 8a

Coumadin blocks factors 2, 7, 9, and 10, which are the vitamin K–dependent coagulation factors. It also blocks proteins C and S, which are responsible for anticoagulation. Thus, the initial effect of Coumadin is to place the patient in a procoagulant state by inhibiting factors C and S.

Question 8b

How do you reverse the effects of Coumadin?

Answer 8b

Coumadin is reversed by administration of vitamin K. For emergency situations, FFP can be given to temporarily replace factors 2, 7, 9, and 10.

Asthma

9. You are paged to the PACU to evaluate an 18-year-old patient complaining of pain after a right inguinal hernia repair under general anesthesia. She has a history of asthma and takes daily Advair.

Question 9a

Could you give this patient ketorolac?

Answer 9a

No, I would not give this patient ketorolac because she has a history of asthma. In general, patients with asthma should not receive NSAIDs given the risk of developing an exacerbation of their asthmatic symptoms.

Question 9b

The patient asks you if she could have had this case performed with an epidural anesthetic. How do you respond?

Answer 9b

Epidural anesthesia is an option for such surgeries, but the decision of whether or not to perform such a technique cannot be made unless a thorough discussion occurs with the surgeon regarding the size and dimensions of the hernia. If this was a small hernia, intense muscle relaxation was not required, and the patient consented to the technique, then an epidural can be a nice option. However, if this was a large hernia that required intense muscle relaxation and/or there were contraindications to an epidural in this patient, then I would not have entertained an epidural approach.

Spinal Technique

10. You are supervising a first-year anesthesia resident as she is performing a spinal anesthetic.

Question 10a

Which ligaments of the back would the resident traverse in trying to reach the epidural space?

Answer 10a

To reach the spinal canal, the resident would traverse the supraspinous, interspinous, and then the ligamentum flavum before reaching the epidural space.

Question 10b

How does the midline approach differ from the paramedian approach?

Answer 10b

In the midline approach, the supraspinous, interspinous, and ligamentum flavum are traversed. However, in the paramedian approach, the needle is inserted not in the midline, but 1–2 cm lateral to the spinous process and only the ligamentum flavum is traversed.

Suggested References

Atchabahian A, Gupta R. *The Anesthesia Guide*. New York: McGraw-Hill; 2013.

Barash PG, Cullen BF, Stoelting RK, Cahalan M, Stock CM, eds. *Clinical Anesthesia*. 6th ed. Philadelphia, PA: Lippincott Williams & Wilkins; 2009.

Horlocker TT, Wedel DJ, Rowlingson JC, et al. Regional anesthesia in the patient receiving antithrombotic or thrombolytic therapy: American Society of Regional Anesthesia and Pain Medicine evidence-based guidelines (third edition). *Reg Anesth Pain Med*. 2010;35:64–101.

39 Additional Topics: Critical Care

Ruchir Gupta

Latex Allergy

1. A 34-year-old female presents for a laparoscopic cholecystectomy. She claims to have a severe anaphylactic allergy to latex.

Question 1a

What precautions would you take in this patient with respect to her latex allergy?

Answer 1a

I would take several precautions in this patient. First, I would make sure all of my anesthesia equipment (injection ports, circuit) are latex free, including the rubber stoppers on the drug vials. If there is any doubt, I would remove the stoppers and draw drugs directly from the vial. I would remove all latex rubber gloves from the OR and use nonpowdered latex-free gloves. I would make sure the OR is clearly marked "latex-free" so that all healthcare providers are aware throughout the case. If possible, I would try to make this the first case of the day, to avoid any contamination from a previous case. Given the nature of the latex allergy, I would have resuscitation drugs handy, including Benadryl, dexamethasone, and epinephrine, in the unlikely event this patient is exposed to latex despite these precautions. I would also have a team meeting with the surgeon and the nurses in the room to ensure they have also made the appropriate adjustments to make sure latex-free equipment is used.

Question 1b

What medical conditions are associated with latex allergies?

Answer 1b

Patients who have worked in the rubber industry or healthcare industry are at risk for latex allergy. Patients with urogenital abnormalities such as spina bifida are also at risk. Patients with an allergy to bananas and kiwi are at risk. Finally, patients who have undergone several surgeries since childhood are at risk.

Hetastarch

2. A 36-year-old female was pulled out of a burning building. She has severe burns to over 50% of her body. The patient is brought to the OR for an emergent repair of an open radius fracture.

Question 2a

Your resident suggests that you use colloid in this patient. How do you respond?

Answer 2a

I would avoid using colloid as the primary fluid in this patient. Burn patients have leaky capillaries, which causes extravasation of proteins from the intravascular space into the extravascular compartment. Exogenous colloids administration would exacerbate this problem by worsening this outward force. Thus, I would opt to give this patient crystalloid.

Question 2b

What are the potential side effects associated with hetastarch?

Answer 2b

Hetastarch has several potential complications, including headache, itching, parotid gland enlargement, anaphylactoid reactions, and coagulation abnormalities such as transient prolongation of PT/PTT and bleeding time.

Fat Embolism Syndrome

3. A 56-year-old homeless man underwent an open reduction internal fixation (ORIF) of an open right femur 2 days ago. He is now in the ICU with signs of respiratory distress.

Question 3a

How is fat embolism syndrome diagnosed?

Answer 3a

To diagnose fat embolism, the Gurd's criteria must be employed. One sign from the major criteria and at least four signs from the minor criteria must be seen in order to make the diagnosis. The major criteria are PaO_2 <60 mmHg, axillary or subconjunctival petechiae, occurring transiently in 50–60% of cases, and CNS depression disproportionate to the hypoxemia. The minor criteria are HR >110 bpm, temperature >38.5°C, emboli in retina, fat in urine, drop in Hct or platelets, increased erythrocyte sedimentation rate (ESR) or plasma viscosity, and fat globules in sputum.

Question 3b

What would you expect a chest X-ray to show in a fat embolism syndrome?

Answer 3b

A chest X-ray routinely shows bilateral infiltrates.

Magnesium Overdose

4. A 34-year-old G1P0 female with pre-eclampsia is receiving magnesium (Mg) therapy.

Question 4a

What are the side effects of magnesium therapy?

Answer 4a

Magnesium therapy is associated with sedation, muscle weakness, cardiac depression, neonatal depression, tocolysis, prolonged labor, and respiratory depression.

Question 4b

What EKG abnormalities are associated with magnesium overdose?

Answer 4b

The cardiac manifestations are different depending on the Mg level. A level between 5 and 8 mEq/L is associated with a prolongation of PR interval and widening of the QRS complex. At 15 mEq/L, one would expect sinoatrial (SA) and atrioventricular (AV) nodal block. At 25 mEq/L one would expect a full-blown cardiac arrest.

Disseminated Intravascular Coagulation (DIC)

5. You are providing general anesthesia for a 45-year-old female who is having an exploratory laparotomy for a ruptured diverticulitis. Midway through the case you notice symptoms of DIC.

Question 5a

How will you respond?

Answer 5a

DIC is a life-threatening emergency. I would call for help and immediately check the vital signs, making sure the patient is oxygenating and ventilating well on 100% O_2. I would open IV fluids wide and establish at least two large-bore IV access (>18 g) to aid in fluid resuscitation. Next, I would administer blood products, including FFP, cryoprecipitate, platelets, and PRBCs, through a rapid transfuser. Depending on the patient's clinical condition, I would place invasive monitors such as an arterial line and a central line to aid in the hemodynamic management of this patient.

Question 5b

What is DIC?

Answer 5b

DIC stands for disseminated intravascular coagulation. As the name implies, blood coagulates within the blood vessels, leading to a consumption of coagulation productions. As a result, massive hemorrhage occurs while thrombosis ensues intravascularly. The net effect is profound anemia, hypovolemia, thrombocytopenia, and hemodynamic instability. If uncorrected, DIC leads to shock and end-organ damage.

Sarcoidosis

6. A 41-year-old female with a history of severe sarcoidosis presents for a right knee replacement.

Question 6a

Would you offer a regional or general technique for this patient?

Answer 6a

Based on the information given, it seems likely that this patient has severe lung disease secondary to her sarcoidosis. Thus, a regional technique will allow me to avoid instrumenting the airway and instituting positive pressure ventilation. A regional technique provides superior analgesia without depressing the respiratory drive. Additionally, given her sarcoidosis, it seems likely that she will have difficulty being weaned off the ventilator.

Question 6b

If you did decide to conduct this case with general anesthesia, can an LMA be used?

Answer 6b

Yes. Depending on the length of the case, an LMA can certainly be used. Sarcoidosis does not increase the risk of aspiration. Additionally, an LMA would allow the patient to maintain spontaneous ventilation throughout the case, which would minimize the amount of respiratory depressant drugs I would have to administer.

Allergic Reactions

7. A 24-year-old female presents for a left foot bunionectomy. During the administration of cefazolin, the patient develops severe hypotension, bronchospasm, and hives over her torso.

Question 7a

What is the mechanism of an anaphylactic reaction?

Answer 7a

It is mediated when the IgE antibody–antigen (cefazolin) complex binds to mast cells, causing them to degranulate. The substances degranulated by mast cells and basophils lead to hypotension, bronchospasm, and, ultimately, full-blown cardiovascular and respiratory collapse.

Question 7b

How does anaphylaxis differ from anaphylactoid reactions?

Answer 7b

In anaphylaxis, an antigen causes the production of IgE antibodies, which bind to mast cells and cause degranulation. In anaphylactoid, the antigen itself binds to the mast cells and causes the degranulation.

Blood Transfusion

8. A 44-year-old Jehovah's Witness presents for a Whipple's procedure. She states she does not want a blood transfusion under any circumstances.

Question 8a

In what circumstances would you avoid using cell saver?

Answer 8a

I would avoid cell saver in conditions that lead to contamination of the surgical field with amniotic fluid, fecal material, tumor cells, Betadine, bone cement, gastric fluids, and epinephrine.

Question 8b

Under what circumstances would you avoid acute normovolemic hemodilution (ANH)?

Answer 8b

I would avoid ANH in any patient who has severe cardiac disease, because anemia will cause an increase in myocardial work and increase the demand side of the supply-and-demand ratio. I would also avoid it in severe renal disease because the extra fluid administered to the patient would need to be effectively excreted by the kidneys. The patient will not be able to get rid of the excess fluid and may develop CHF and electrolyte abnormalities. Finally, I would avoid it in conditions where the patient's baseline Hb is already low (<11 g/dL).

Aspiration

9. You are performing general anesthesia with an LMA on a 63-year-old patient who is having right knee arthroscopy.

Question 9a

Midway through the case, you notice the patient is coughing and her oropharynx is filled with the Bicitra you gave her preoperatively for her GERD. How do you respond?

Answer 9a

I would immediately remove the LMA, suction the oropharynx, put the back of the head up, and emergently intubate the patient. I would ventilate with 100% O_2 and auscultate the chest for any abnormal breath sounds. I would add PEEP to the ventilator and administer a beta-agonist nebulizer as needed. I would assess the BP and heart rate and consider opening the fluids wide and treating the hypotension with a pressor. Finally, I would ask that a chest X-ray be done in the PACU.

Question 9b

The case continues uneventfully and the patient is easily extubated. Will you discharge this patient home as planned or admit her for an overnight stay at the hospital?

Answer 9b

It depends on the course of her surgery. If the patient continued to show no signs of respiratory distress for 2 hours in the PACU and her breath sounds were clear to auscultation with a normal-appearing chest X-ray, I would allow her to be discharged with follow-up to her medical doctor. If, however, she was desaturating in the PACU and/or had wheezing and needed beta-agonist therapy, I would admit her for overnight stay and consider consulting the pulmonary service.

TPN

10. A 64-year-old homeless man was found unresponsive by the emergency medical service (EMS). He is currently in the ICU and is receiving total parenteral nutrition (TPN) via a central line.

Question 10a

What is refeeding syndrome?

Answer 10a

Refeeding syndrome is a syndrome of electrolyte imbalances that is seen when a patient receives TPN therapy after a period of starvation. Patients with anorexia, kwashiorkor, marasmus, and chronic alcoholism are at greatest risk. The electrolyte abnormalities most commonly seen are hypophosphatemia, hypokalemia, hypomagnesemia, glucose imbalance, vitamin deficiency, and fluid imbalance.

Question 10b

What other complications of TPN would you be wary of?

Answer 10b

TPN therapy is associated with bacterial infection, fatty liver, venous thrombosis, metabolic acidosis, and hypercarbia.

Suggested References

Atchabahian A, Gupta, R, eds. *The Anesthesia Guide*. New York: McGraw Hill; 2013.

Miller RD, Eriksson LI, Fleisher LA, Wiener-Kornish JP, Young WL, eds. *Miller's Anesthesia*. 7th ed. Philadelphia, PA: Churchill Livingstone Elsevier; 2010.

II Applied Examination: The OSCE

1 Basics of Objective Structured Clinical Exam (OSCE)

William Vuong and Ruchir Gupta

One of the most exciting developments in anesthesiology education has been the introduction of simulators as learning tools. The use of simulation in medical education has only become vogue relatively recently, with anesthesiology as a specialty providing a strong voice for its inclusion in training. Supporters cite increased patient safety as well as the ability to teach responses to situations that are either too rare or dangerous for daily anesthesia practice.

The American Board of Anesthesiology (ABA) has decided to include simulations within a broader structure of an OSCE where the simulations are not just with robots and computers but also with live patients.

This portion of the exam is divided into two parts—communication and professionalism, and technical skills related to patient care. The student is required to participate in a seven-station circuit that will evaluate his or her proficiency in seven of the nine skills listed in the OSCE Content Outline. Each OSCE is 8 minutes long with 4 minutes between stations to review the next scenario. The OSCE portion of the APPLIED Exam takes 84 minutes from start to finish.

In some exam rooms, candidates will interact with a standardized patient actor while in others they will interact directly with an examiner, but examiners will not be in most exam rooms. In such circumstances, the sessions will be recorded for grading purposes.

Because the technical skills portion is difficult to learn from a book, our focus here is exclusively on the first six scenarios that focus on communication and professionalism. For the three possible scenarios on the technical skills portion, the reader should visit the ABA website, at www.theaba.org, and view the online simulations.

2 Clinical Scenario #1: Informed Consent

John Smith is a 55-year-old patient who is scheduled for a left knee arthroplasty. The patient reports stiffness and pain in the knee for the past 6 months and has been advised that a knee replacement is his best option. The patient was evaluated last week in the preoperative evaluation clinic and your colleague has approved the patient for anesthesia.

Past medical history is significant for hypertension and hypercholesterolemia. Hb is 11.3 g/dL. The EKG is normal. There is no evidence of heart disease. Review of symptoms is otherwise negative.

Medications include lisinopril (last dose yesterday) and Zocor.
Prior surgical history includes a right inguinal hernia repair.
Physical exam is unremarkable, with a class I airway.
Vital signs are HR 85 bpm; BP 148/84 mmHg.
The patient has no allergies.
The patient is appropriately NPO.

The patient has already agreed to proceed with general anesthesia after speaking with your colleague who will be providing general anesthesia in the operating room. Your anesthesia group also routinely offers a peripheral nerve block as part of the anesthetic plan for knee surgery. The block is performed preoperatively by a separate regional anesthesiology team that you are leading today. You agree that regional analgesia is appropriate in this patient. A separate informed consent for general anesthesia has already been obtained by your colleague.

Task Statement

Your task is to obtain informed consent for the nerve block. Your institution does not employ written informed consent (verbal consent is sufficient). You should NOT repeat your colleague's history and physical examination.

Action Plan

For this particular scenario, the ABA wishes to have the student address the following eight points: (1) why the procedure is needed; (2) conducting of the procedure in lay terms; (3) the benefits and risks of the procedure, including both less severe/more common and more severe/less common material risks; (4) alternatives (if appropriate); (5) identifying all persons participating in the procedure; (6) demonstration of ability to elicit questions and respond appropriately in lay terms; (7) demonstration of ability to elicit affirmative consent without coercion; and (8) understanding of and concern for the situation of the patient.

Step 1: Identify the Medicine behind the Question

In this scenario, the student must first determine which block is most appropriate for knee surgery. While knee surgery can be performed with a spinal or epidural, the scenario specifies that your team is planning for a peripheral nerve block, not a neuraxial. Thus, the possibilities are limited to a femoral nerve block or, less commonly, an adductor canal block. KEEP IT SIMPLE. The OSCE is not your opportunity to overly impress the ABA with the most cutting edge technique. The purpose is merely to assess baseline level of confidence so it is advisable to use the most commonly used block and/or a block that you frequently have done and are comfortable discussing. Here we will use the femoral nerve block.

The femoral nerve block provides innervation to the anterior two-thirds of the knee, but the posterior one-third is not innervated by the femoral nerve. Thus, this information must be explained to the patient.

Step 2: Approach the Patient

Always begin this portion by introducing yourself and shaking the patient's hand.

> "Hello, Mr. Smith. I'm Dr. Gupta, one of the anesthesiologists at this hospital. How are you?"

It's usually important to initially provide a brief description before you delve into your specific role within the anesthesia department. After the initial statement, look at the hospital ID band and say:

> "Can you tell me your full name and date of birth? . . . Thank you, and what procedure are you having?"

Now that you have confirmed that this is indeed the correct patient and that he is having the surgery that is listed on the schedule, delve into the details of your role:

> "So, for this type of procedure, we have the patient go to sleep. However, we are concerned about your pain after the surgery when you wake up. So, we like to perform what is known as a nerve block. I am the head of the 'nerve block team' today."

Notice the lay terms being used (*so*, not *hence* or *thus*). Keep in mind you are talking to an everyday person, not a medical professional. Avoid terminology such as *analgesia* or *postoperative*, instead using words such as *pain* and *after surgery*.

At this point, you have established rapport with the patient, confirmed that this is the correct patient and procedure, and introduced your role in his care. This step should not take more than 1 minute of your time and is essential to establishing you as a thorough and caring provider to the examiners.

Step 3: Begin Completing Tasks

We already began addressing task #1 (why the procedure is needed) during the previous step by introducing to the patient that he will have considerable pain after surgery. However, now that rapport has been establish, it is time to be more focused:

> "The specific procedure I would like to perform is called a 'femoral nerve block.' Basically, nerves come off of our spinal cord and go to different parts of our body. For the knee, there is a large nerve called the 'femoral' which wraps over to the front of our body near the groin and moves further down to our knee. By depositing some local anesthesia around this nerve, you will basically have no feeling on the front two-thirds of your knee for a good 8–12 hours. You will still have feeling on the back of your knee because a different nerve goes there, but we can try to control that pain with some pills. The benefit here is that the front two-thirds should be pain free."

Here we have fully addressed task #1 and begun to discuss task #2 (conducting of procedure in lay terms). However, we must be more detail oriented in order to get full credit for task #2. It is unclear if the "patient" in these scenarios will ask questions that will elicit the student to move on to the next task. It is advised that if the patient does not ask questions, it would be prudent to simply keep talking in a stepwise manner, addressing task #1 to task #8. Here we will proceed as if the patient is asking questions:

> Patient: Ok, so where are we going to do this?
>
> Student: We will do it right here because this area is actually called the "block area." First, I will clean the area where we are going to inject the medicine with a special chemical to kill any bacteria. Then, using sterile gloves and sterile equipment, we will put on a little drape. I will use an ultrasound machine to locate the nerve and, once I see it, I will introduce a small needle into the area and under direct visualization I will inject a small dose of local anesthesia.
>
> Next, go directly into the risks and benefits, because it flows well:
>
> "Risks involved with this procedure include the risk of infection. Thus, I will use only sterile equipment and will also use a special prep to clean the area. There is also a risk of bleeding because we are going near blood vessels. To minimize this risk, we are using an ultrasound machine so that we can see exactly where our needle is. I will also be pulling back on my syringe before injecting because if I am in a blood vessel, blood will return into my syringe. There is also a risk of nerve damage if we inject directly into the nerve. Thus, the ultrasound machine will assist us in avoiding this risk. Lastly, there is a risk that the local anesthesia is

injected directly into the blood vessel, which can be very toxic. Both my pulling back on the syringe prior to injection and my use of the ultrasound machine will help me avoid this."

Again, notice how technical terms such as *aspirating* and *catheter* have been replaced with "pull back," and "needle." As you mention the risks, immediately go to the precautionary steps you will take to minimize the risk. This provides the patient with immediate reinforcement so that he is not provided with a litany of terrible possibilities. Consider the following example:

"Risks involved include infection, bleeding, nerve damage, and possible cardiac arrest."

This would be an example of an incomplete, nonempathic answer which will likely confuse the patient and lead him to not consent.

It is now important to say that there are alternatives (task #4). Here, we assume the patient has not stated anything and is just listening to you:

"There are alternatives to this procedure. I can give you pain medication through your IV. However, this may not provide as much pain relief as the nerve block because they work by a different mechanism. Additionally, the medications I would administer would likely include narcotics, which are associated with side effects such as nausea and vomiting, itching, and constipation. The benefit of these drugs is that I could just give them to you while you are asleep, with no additional needle sticks, but the downside is that they are associated with some undesirable side effects and the pain may not be as well controlled."

Do NOT go into an evidenced-based doctrine on different studies and what different researchers have found. Keep it simple, using terms such as *likely* and *possibly* and attempt to not "sell" one approach over another. Simply state pros and cons and be clear.

On to task #5 (identify all persons participating in the procedure):

"I would perform the block myself but I will have the nurse adjust my ultrasound machine. I also have a resident who may assist me with some aspects of the procedure. At all times, your safety will be my number one priority."

This is your chance to introduce safety. Notice this has not been identified by the ABA content outline as one of the tasks. However, ensuring patient safety is a fundamental goal of patient care, and by proactively introducing it, you are ahead of the curve.

Task #6 (demonstration of ability to elicit questions and respond appropriately in lay terms):

"Do you have any questions about anything that I told you?"

Ask a very open-ended question that makes it clear the patient is not restricted to specific aspects of your talk, such as the actual procedure, or who is performing it, or the risks. Here is your opportunity to make a clear, all-inclusive statement. It is also important to pause here to allow the patient to process the information provided so that he does not feel rushed. Lastly, be sure of what you have presented because there are limitless questions that can be asked. Because each scenario lasts only 8 minutes, the patient will likely not ask too many questions, if any.

On to task #7 (demonstration of ability to elicit affirmative consent without coercion):

"Would it be ok if we proceeded with the nerve block?"

Because the scenario is nudging you to obtain consent for the block, it is advisable to not provide a totally open-ended question here. Examples of an improper question for task #7 are as follows:

"Would you rather not do the block?"—too suggestive of alternative

"Do you want to proceed with the block or the IV pain medications instead?"—too open-ended

"Have the nurse page me if you decide to do the block."—too dismissive

Now that we have completed the first seven tasks, the only task left is a largely nontechnical one: understanding of and concern for the situation of the patient (task #8). Often this task will be completed when you ask the patient if he has any questions. It is not advisable to repeat your response if it was already provided there. However, to ensure that you completed task #8 during the question period, you should use some buzzwords. Consider the following examples:

Task 6:

Student: Do you have any questions about anything that I told you?

Patient: I'm scared about needles while I'm awake.

Student: I can understand the *concerns* you have for this situation. Having someone inject a needle can sometimes be terrifying even for us doctors. One thing I can do for you is that before I do anything, I will give you a small dose of a drug called Versed. You will feel like you have had a few martinis. This would put you more at ease. Then, before I do anything I will tell you so there are no surprises. Would this make this *situation* less worrisome to you?

Notice the emphasis on the words *concern* and *situation*. They are coming straight out of the content outline! Thus, a reviewer of the video can easily determine that this task (task #8) has been adequately addressed and will ensure complete points. Following is an example of a response that would garner credit for task #6 but may not earn the points for task #8.

Task #6:

Student: Do you have any questions about anything that I told you.?

Patient: I'm scared about needles while I'm awake.

Student: Everybody is. This is a normal response. We can offer you sedation if you like so you are not so anxious.

This response fails to really show empathy and concern for the patient's situation. Comparing this to the previous response, the student doesn't talk about how doctors also feel this way or how sedation makes a patient feel (drunk with martinis), and it seems overly brief and technical (i.e., sedation may mean different things to different nonmedical individuals).

In summary, the pillars of informed consent are to show empathy, be thorough but use nontechnical language, be brief, and be up front about alternatives. While there is a clear bias that the clinician has about what is the best choice, it is important to present the pros and cons of the procedure and the alternatives and provide an opportunity for a discussion. Of all of the aforementioned tasks, it is the use of nontechnical language that students struggle with most, as they are not used to discussing medicine with nonclinicians. It is good to avoid terms such as *analgesia, postoperative*, and *sedation*.

3 Clinical Scenario #2: Treatment Options

Jane Smith is a 35-year-old patient who lacerated multiple tendons in her hand when she accidentally smashed a glass vase while trying to clean it. She has not eaten or drunk anything since early this morning (>8 hours ago).

Past medical history is significant for her mother dying of a fever during a hernia repair. The patient was told that she may be susceptible to the same type of fever. The patient does not smoke or drink and has no other medical concerns.

The patient takes no medications.

The patient is a professional distance runner.

Physical exam shows normal airway and cardiopulmonary exams. Vital signs are BP 115/65 mmHg, HR 66 bpm, SpO_2 99%, pain score 5 out of 10. She has no allergies.

You are the attending anesthesiologist seeing the patient in the preoperative holding area. A resident working with you has already completed the preoperative evaluation. However, the patient has concerns about both general and regional anesthesia related to experiences of her mother and asks to speak to you about options.

Task Statement

Your task is to discuss with the patient the anesthetic options given the patient's specific concerns and agree upon an anesthetic plan. You should NOT repeat the history and physical examination and do NOT need to obtain formal informed consent, which will be obtained by the anesthesia resident after your discussion.

Action Plan

For this particular scenario, the ABA wishes to have the student address the following five points: (1) relevant treatment options; (2) risks and benefits of options; (3) ability to question and respond appropriately in lay terms; (4) confirm final decision regarding treatment choice with the patient; (5) demonstrate understanding of and concern for the situation of the patient.

Step 1: Identify the Medicine behind the Question

In this scenario, the student must first recognize that the "fever" being referred to is most likely malignant hyperthermia (MH). While knowing the specific mechanism at the molecular level is beyond the scope of this exam, the student must identify the causes (triggers) of MH and how it can be avoided. Additionally, the student must also be aware of what treatment options will minimize this risk and if, despite all precautions taken, the patient develops MH, how the student will treat the condition.

Step 2: Approach the Patient

Always begin this portion by introducing yourself and shaking her hand:

> "Hello, Ms. Smith. I'm Dr. Gupta, one of the anesthesiologists at this hospital. How are you?"

It's usually important to initially provide a brief description before you delve into your specific role within the anesthesia department. After the initial statement, look at her hospital ID band and say:

> "Can you tell me your full name and date of birth? . . . Thank you, and what procedure are you having?"

Now that you have confirmed that this is indeed the correct patient and that she is having the surgery that is listed on the schedule, delve into the tasks.

Step 3: Begin Completing Tasks

To begin the discussion about choice of anesthetic you might start with the following:

> "My resident informed me of your family member's experience with anesthesia in the past and I wanted to discuss with you some options that can allow more safety for you for this case."

Using the word *safety* is crucial here, because it highlights the fact that you are engaging in good patient care and offering the patient safe options for her anesthesia.

To address task #1, it must be understood that the patient's anesthesia care can be broadly categorized into two possibilities: regional with sedation or general with total intravenous anesthesia (TIVA). Keep in mind that the simpler your choice, the easier the exam will be. There is no benefit to try something you are not familiar with (e.g., dexmedetomidine infusion). The choice for regional may be several different blocks, but infraclavicular is likely the best option. Also, if you are going to suggest a block, make sure you know the risks and benefits associated with it.

> "It seems you have a possible susceptibility to a condition known as malignant hyperthermia, which can be fatal. To avoid this, we can do this case one of two ways: I could have you to go to sleep with a breathing tube and use anesthesia drugs that do not cause this condition. These drugs would just flow in through your IV and you would not receive any anesthetic gases. The other option is to perform an infraclavicular block. In this a procedure I would deposit a small amount of local anesthetic around the nerves that go to your hand. Your hand would be

numb and I would give you sleepy medicine during the case. The difference here is that there would be no breathing tube and you would be breathing on your own."

Notice the use of lay terms (*deposit* vs. *inject, gases* vs. *volatile anesthetics, breathing tube* vs. *intubation*). Also, notice how TIVA anesthesia is explained in a manner that a nonanesthesiologist may be able to understand. Consider the following example of an inadequate response:

"It seems you are susceptible to a condition known as malignant hyperthermia. Thus, I would avoid triggering agents and likely use the TIVA technique. I could also do a block with some sedation if you prefer."

While this response may seem understandable to most anesthesiologists, the purpose of these scenarios is mainly to ascertain if you can communicate effectively with nonmedical personnel about medical choices.

It is unclear if at this point your patient will prompt you to discuss the risks and benefits of each technique (task #2). If you do not receive a prompt, simply continue, since that would also be your normal conversation flow.

"There are risks and benefits of each technique. With the general approach, where you have a breathing tube, you will be completely asleep and unaware of what is happening. The downside is that you will need pain medication, which I would then provide through your IV. These medications include narcotics, which have the side effect of nausea, itching, and constipation. The other disadvantage is that you are on the ventilator, and if there is any minor trace amount of gases that cause MH, you may become exposed. The benefits of the regional technique are that the nerves going to your arm are completely numb and this numbness lasts for a good 8–12 hours, so the pain relief is great. Additionally, I would just have you breath oxygen through your nose and you would not be connected to a ventilator. The risk, however, is that the nerve block itself can have complications, such as infection, bleeding, and possible lung injury, since I am going near your lung."

There is a fair amount of information that must be covered for task #2, but if you are organized, it will flow clearly and your response will be thorough. For task #3, you have to open the floor for questions and be prepared for just about any question. Odds are that the patient will ask very basic questions. Consider the possible example:

Patient: Which technique lowers my risk of MH more?

Student: Both techniques protect equally. However, because we use the so-called MH-triggering agents routinely in our ventilator, there is a slight chance that some trace element may remain in the ventilator if we do general. Again, I highly doubt that will happen, because I will flush the ventilator thoroughly with oxygen as per protocol and I do not believe we will have any trace elements left. However, there is certainly no way to guarantee this.

Do not make up facts. If neither technique has been proven to be more efficacious in preventing MH, then do not simply state this just to further your own bias. Remember, this portion of the test is less about the "what" and more about the "how." Thus, notice the choice of words in the previous statement ("I highly doubt," "certainly no way").

For task #4 (confirms final decision regarding treatment choice with the patient), it is important to show empathy to the patient given her situation and to ask the question appropriately.

"Do you know how would you like us to proceed?"

Notice how we are framing the final decision with a question. There are inappropriate ways of ascertaining the final decision which must be avoided:

"So, tell me what you want to do."—abrasive

"Shall I get the nerve block team for you?"—suggestive

"If I were you, I would go with the nerve block."—coercive

Task #5 will likely be accomplished during the question-and-answer portion of the OSCE (task #3). It is important to use the words *concern* and *understand* in your response as this will help the examiner recognize that you are addressing this task and you will receive the appropriate credit. If, however, you feel that this task has not been adequately addressed in the course of the exam, it would be prudent to end with the following statement:

> "I know how *concerned* you must be. I understand your situation completely and I assure you I will do everything possible to make sure we do not administer any agent that can cause MH. We have some terrific new drugs since the time of your mom's surgery that can help us get through the procedure without the need for any of the agents that led to your mom developing her fever. I will make sure that we use the right agents and I will have all of my backup emergency equipment ready and available so if you do somehow show signs of MH, we can rapidly treat it."

The details of the treatment are not relevant here. Simply mentioning that you will exercise your due diligence in avoiding triggering agents and have "back up emergency equipment" ready (i.e., MH cart) is adequate for the lay person.

In summary, discussions about treatment options must be presented as pros and cons and explained at a level that a lay person can understand. In preparing for this scenario, the student should practice how to explain certain topics such as TIVA, regional, neuraxial, blood transfusion, anaphylaxis, and MH, using a layperson's terminology. Each of these topics is high yield and will possibly show up on the exam.

4 Clinical Scenario #3: Periprocedural Complications

You provided general anesthesia for Jane Doe, an otherwise healthy patient who received a laparoscopic inguinal herniorrhaphy. Although Jane Doe has an allergy to cephalosporins, you accidentally administered 2 grams of cefoxitin prior to incision. Despite this, the patient had no alteration in hemodynamics and the surgery went well. You informed the surgeon of this incident as it happened and a decision was made to have the crash cart in the room in case the patient developed any signs of an allergic reaction. Additionally, you both agreed the patient should be admitted to the hospital and observed overnight before being discharged home. The patient is now awake, alert, and comfortable in the PACU. The surgeon has informed the patient that there was a medication error, and that you will be discussing this error with the patient.

Task Statement

Your task is to discuss this medication error with the patient.

Action Plan

For this particular scenario, the ABA wishes to have the student address the following seven points: (1) elicit history relevant to the complication and current symptoms; (2) perform a focused physical evaluation, if appropriate; (3) discuss potential causes; (4) discuss potential outcomes; (5) present a plan for further evaluation and/or treatment, if appropriate; (6) elicit questions and responses appropriately in lay terms; and (7) demonstrate understanding of and concern for the situation of the patient.

Step 1: Identify the Medicine behind the Question

Allergic reactions can be of multiple types: febrile, nonhemolytic, hemolytic, and anaphylactic. When a patient with an allergy to a drug—in this case, an antibiotic—presents for medical evaluation, it is crucial to ascertain what specifically occurs upon exposure to the offending agent (i.e., rash, difficulty breathing, etc.).

In this scenario, we are limited in our understanding of the nature of this allergy and are simply told the patient has an "allergy" to cephalosporins, and yet a drug of this class was administered. Despite this, no signs of an allergic reaction developed. Thus, we are left to wonder whether this is even a true allergy. It is important to know that you are not an immunologist and the absence of any symptoms upon exposure cannot be used to conclude that the patient has no allergies to cephalosporins. For this, the patient must go to an immunology clinic and undergo allergy testing.

Step 2: Approach the Patient

Always begin this portion by introducing yourself and shaking the patient's hand:

> "Hello, Ms. Doe. It's Dr. Gupta, your anesthesiologist. How are you feeling?"

Recall that this patient is positioned in the PACU after receiving an anesthetic. Thus, you are not theoretically meeting her for the first time (though in actuality you are meeting the actor for the first time). Begin by asking a general question about how the patient is feeling, just as you would if you approached a patient in the PACU.

Step 3: Begin Completing Tasks

Begin with task #1 (elicit history relevant to the complication and current symptoms):

> "I had some questions regarding your allergy to cephalosporins. Could you tell me when you were first told you were allergic to these drugs?"

Start with an open-ended question. It is hard to say what the patient will say at this point. She may give you a thorough recollection of a previous surgery, or that all of her relatives were allergic so she always thought she was as well, or even say that she didn't know she had the allergy but her doctor told her she did. Thus, you may need some more follow-up questions based on her response:
True anaphylactic allergy:

> Patient: I had my gallbladder out a few years ago and the anesthesiologist told me my blood pressure had dropped and I stopped breathing as soon as they gave me that drug.

True nonanaphylactic reaction:

> Patient: I once took it and broke out in hives all over my body.

Nonallergic reaction mislabeled as an allergy:

> Patient: I once had my primary doctor give me one of those pills and I just kept vomiting, so I assumed I was allergic.
>
> In each of these scenarios, the response will be:
>
> Student: I see. And was that the only time you have ever been exposed to that drug?

Now explain to the patient the exact event and provide reassurance immediately:

"The reason I'm asking you this is because as your surgeon probably mentioned, you were accidentally given a dose of a cephalosporin, but fortunately, your vital signs remained stable the entire time and there were no issues at all. We are very pleased actually with the outcome and how it seemed to us that your body did not react in any adverse way to the dose. However, now that you are awake I wanted to ask you some more detailed questions about how your feeling."

Now your questions should focus more on the present, in the form of a focused history of current symptoms (task #2, perform focused physical evaluation if appropriate):

"Are you currently experiencing any shortness of breath or difficulty breathing?" (Respiratory)

"Do you have any light-headedness or chest tightness or discomfort?" (Cardiovascular)

"How is your belly? Any abnormal pain or sensation?" (GI)

"Do you have any itching or hives anywhere that you noticed?"

Now that you have completed your history, do a physical (task #2) by FIRST evaluating the vital signs (HR, BP, RR, temperature). If a thermometer is not available, you should verbalize:

"I think the nurse took my thermometer. I will ask her what your most recent temperature was."

This way the examiner knows you wanted to obtain a temperature, which is crucial for a patient with an exposure to a suspected allergic agent.

Then, listen to the heart and lungs. Ask the patient to open her mouth, and evaluate the tongue and oropharynx for any sores (HEENT exam). Look at the patient's arms, legs, and back to evaluate for the presence of any hives.

For task #3 (potential causes) and task #4 (potential outcomes), begin with a general discussion of what you think happened.

"So, like I said, you did receive a cephalosporin during this surgery, but nothing during your anesthetic or now during my physical exam is telling me that you have any signs of an allergic reaction. I still would want to keep you here overnight just so we can keep a close eye to make sure nothing develops, but most of the time the allergic reaction will be immediate and not take several hours to develop, at least with this type of an allergy."

If the patient wants more information, she may ask:

Patient: What might you expect to see if something does develop later on tonight?

Student: To be honest, I don't expect to see any issues with breathing or blood pressure this far out. That being said, anything you experience out of the ordinary will automatically be thought to be possibly from this exposure, so it is important to be able to keep a close eye on things.

Keep in mind throughout this OSCE that you are not being graded on your understanding of the medicine or even your management, but instead your completion of the tasks—tasks which are focused more on communication and presentation than on hard facts. That being said, using terms such as *possibly* or *most likely* will protect you from being docked points for inaccurate statements.

For task #5 (plan for further evaluation and/or treatment), you can begin utilizing consults, as we are now approaching areas of medicine that are not in your specialty:

> "After we send you home, I will give the number of an immunologist that you can contact who can test you further to see if you do indeed have an allergy to these drugs. I will also have that immunologist say "hi" to you while you are in the hospital."

On to task #6 (elicit questions and responds appropriately in lay terms):

> "Do you have any questions about anything that I told you?"

Ask a very open-ended question that allows the patient to question any aspect of what has been discussed. Keep in mind there are limitless questions that can be asked. Because each scenario lasts only 8 minutes, the patient will likely not ask too many questions, if any.

For task #7 (demonstrate understanding of and concern for the situation of the patient), most of the time this task is intertwined in how you performed the previous six tasks. However, if you still feel the need to show more concern you can end with the following statement:

> "I know this whole incident is very concerning. I just want you to know that we are taking every precaution to make sure you receive the best care and make a safe recovery."

This scenario may seem more daunting than it actually is. The key to doing well for this OSCE is to recognize what type of history and physical you need to do and what type of follow-up care is needed. If the patient presented is an outpatient who had surgery days ago, then admitting that patient to the hospital is not an appropriate choice. In many circumstances, ordering a few follow-up tests and then referring to an expert is acceptable.

5 Clinical Scenario #4: Ethical Issues

You are working in the operating room on call and have just started your clinical shift. Your first patient of the day is John Doe, a patient with suspected ruptured diverticulum who requires an urgent exploratory laparotomy. The patient has multiple serious comorbidities, including metastatic melanoma, coronary artery disease, and poorly controlled hypertension. In the past, the patient has expressed wishes to not be resuscitated and a do not resuscitate (DNR) status has been in place for 1 month. The patient has both medical and cardiac clearance on the chart. Current vital signs are HR 99 bpm, BP 145/75 mmHg, RR 22, SaO_2 96% on room air, pain score of 4 out of 10. The operating room is almost ready for the patient to come back, and you will be providing anesthesia. You have determined that endotracheal intubation is required as a part of the anesthetic plan. The patient has asked specifically to discuss DNR status with you as the anesthesiologist who will care for the patient.

Task Statement

Your task is to discuss how to manage the patient's DNR status in the perioperative period. You do NOT need to obtain formal informed consent for general anesthesia or discuss other aspects of anesthetic care not related to DNR status.

Action Plan

For this particular scenario, the ABA wishes to have the student demonstrate behaviors consistent with application of the principles in the ASA Guideline for the Ethical Practice of Anesthesiology, including the principles of (1) patient autonomy, (2) beneficence, and (3) nonmaleficence.

Step 1: Identify the Medicine behind the Question

Because this is an ethical dilemma question, there is not much in the way of medical physiology that must be known here. However, what one must know is that there are three main options for any DNR patient undergoing anesthesia: (1) rescind the DNR completely during the perioperative course, (2) maintain the DNR that is currently in place, or (3) modify the DNR.

In mostly all situations, option #3 of modifying the DNR is adopted. The modification is simply that if there is an anesthesia-induced, reversible cause of hypotension and/or arrhythmias, then resuscitative measures will be employed. However, if the patient goes into full-blown arrest or it appears that the patient's condition is not reversible, then resuscitative measures will be suspended.

Step 2: Approach the Patient

Always begin this portion by introducing yourself and shaking the patient's hand:

> "Hello, I'm Dr. Gupta, one of the anesthesiologists at this hospital. How are you?"

It's usually important to initially provide a brief description before you delve into your specific role within the anesthesia department. After the initial statement, look at the patient's hospital ID band and say:

> "Can you tell me your full name and date of birth? . . . Thank you, and what procedure are you having?"

Now, that you have confirmed that this is indeed the correct patient and that he is having the surgery that is listed on the schedule, delve into the tasks.

Step 3: Begin Completing Tasks

Now begin by asking the patient about the issue at hand:

> "I understand you wanted to speak to me?"

At this point, the patient will likely bring up his concerns regarding the DNR order (task #1). It is important to nod and appear empathetic while the patient is speaking. Always make eye contact and ensure that you seem as if you are actively listening (though you already know what the issue is).

Once the patient is finished, it is important to present the three options (task #2) in a clear manner:

> "There are three choices that we have here in light of your DNR order. The first is to keep it completely in place. The second is to put it on hold completely during your care. The third, and this is what is usually done and I would also recommend, is to modify your DNR order. By modify, what I mean is that if during your care your blood pressure should drop from a cause that is reversible, I would like to treat you. If, however, your blood pressure drops and the cause is not reversible, I would cease any resuscitation efforts. I would also like to point out that the drugs we give you for anesthesia actually drop your blood pressure as a side effect. So, it is certainly not uncommon for me to give my patients some type of medicine to bring the blood pressure up. I just wanted to be clear about the situations in which I would act."

For the lay person, this answer is quite loaded with information. Thus, the patient may ask questions based on such an answer:

Patient: Doc, I'm really sick and I don't want any CPR. How does this blood pressure stuff fit in with the heart?

Student: Good question. When the blood pressure drops dramatically, the heart has to work extra hard, which means it is at risk of basically giving out. We agree that we shouldn't do CPR and let you go if your heart stops. The gray area here is that if I tell you that I will be giving you a medication which in almost everyone stops their heart, but if I do some maneuvers—not CPR—but give medications through your IV, I can restore your heart rate and blood pressure—do I have your permission to do that?

Much of the discourse for this scenario will center around the patient's questions regarding the issue of resuscitation. It is important to be clear to the patient that resuscitation need not mean chest compressions, but also the administration of a pressor (phenylephrine/ephedrine), fluids, or blood products.

Compared to other scenarios, this particular OSCE is somewhat brief. The best method of preparing for this situation is to speak in layperson's terms and clearly delineate options for the patient. Active listening by making eye contact and appearing empathetic helps.

6 Clinical Scenario #5: Communication with Other Health Professionals

You are scheduled to provide anesthesia for a 62-year-old patient for an elective right inguinal hernia repair under general anesthesia. When you evaluate the patient in the preoperative area, you find that the patient has bilateral wheezing. The patient states that she has a history of emphysema but does not usually experience wheezing. The pulmonary clearance report also indicates that breath sounds were clear bilaterally during the office visit. No other testing or laboratory work is available. Vital signs are BP 105/67 mmHg, HR 77 bpm, RR 23, oxygen saturation 95% on room air. In your clinical judgment, this elective procedure MUST be postponed so that the patient can be treated for the wheezing and be optimized for surgery, if necessary. You will meet with Dr. Joseph Smith, the surgeon who scheduled the case, prior to the start of the case to discuss your concerns.

Task Statement

Your task is to present your recommendation to Dr. Smith to postpone the surgery and determine the best course of action. The discussion is taking place in a consultation room shortly before the scheduled start of the case. You will NOT have any direct interactions with the patient as part of this scenario.

Action Plan

For this particular scenario, the ABA wishes to have the student complete the following tasks: (1) communicate in a clear and professional manner; (2) prioritize communication of information most relevant to patient care; (3) demonstrate understanding of the concerns and perspective of other health care professionals through active listening; and (4) recognize the potential for conflict and initiate conflict resolution as appropriate.

Step 1: Identify the Medicine behind the Question

There are limitless disease states that can be asked about during this simulation. The most common are likely going to be cardiac, pulmonary, or both.

In a patient with emphysema, the presence of wheezing may not seem abnormal. However, two things to be considered here are (1) what is the patient's baseline, and (2) can the patient be optimized before being operated on. In this scenario, there was no wheezing documented on the pulmonary clearance report, and even the patient states not usually experiencing it. Thus, this is a departure from baseline.

Whether the patient can be optimized if the surgery is postponed depends on the cause. In this scenario, the patient may be developing a respiratory infection, or the patient's emphysema may have deteriorated since the last office visit. It is acceptable to defer management to the specialist because it is not suggested here that as the anesthesiologist you must know the exact treatment for a pulmonary condition. Rather, simply sending the patient back to the pulmonologist with a note would suffice.

Step 2: Approach the Surgeon

Always begin this portion by introducing yourself and shaking the colleague's hand:

> "Hi, Dr. Smith. I'm Dr. Gupta. I am scheduled to be in your hernia case."

Step 3: Begin Completing Tasks

Next, communicate your concerns about this patient's case:

> "I have some concerns about your next patient. The patient has bilateral wheezing and decreased breath sounds, and according to the pulmonary note and the patient herself, both these things are new onset. I'm worried this could be an exacerbation of her COPD or that she is beginning to develop a respiratory infection. I don't think she is optimized for surgery."

Here you have clearly stated in one to two sentences what your concerns are, based on the history and physical, and what could be a possible cause of these symptoms (task #1). Notice how we are not focusing here on other portions of the history and physical, but rather just on the pertinent positives.

The surgeon actor can say anything at this point, but likely will express frustration at the delay. The response has to be basically a reiteration of the concern just stated, but a little more detailed. For the purpose of discussion let's suppose the surgeon's response to your statement is as follows:

> Surgeon: Most patients with COPD develop some wheezing from time to time. She doesn't have a fever. Can't you just give her an albuterol treatment?
>
> Student: My concern here is that according to her pulmonology note, this was not the case during the office visit, so it appears to be new onset. Additionally, I could give a few puffs of albuterol, but there's no guarantee that that will fix her wheezing. In her current state, she is at high risk for pulmonary complications during anesthesia and may be difficult to wean off the ventilator.

Here the response goes into greater detail, prioritizing the information (task #2) most relevant to the situation. We first discuss that it is new onset, which means there is likely room for improvement with the right intervention as the patient's baseline consists of no wheezing. We also address the albuterol suggestion, and conclude with discussing the anesthetic complication we are concerned about as a result of this clinical picture.

Surgeon: My concern is that she doesn't stop smoking, and every time we bring her to get her hernia repaired, there is some issue that comes up. She needs her hernia to be repaired.

Student: I understand your concern. However, unless this is an emergency case, I would like to send her to her pulmonologist and ensure that her wheezing is under control before we proceed with a general anesthetic.

It is important at this stage to show empathy for the surgeon's concern (task #3). However, in doing so, basic principles of patient care cannot be compromised. Unless the case is emergent, there is no clinical indication to proceed with the procedure as planned.

The surgeon may respond as follows:

Surgeon: I'm going to ask for another anesthesiologist. We do these patients all the time. This patient has no fever and this makes no sense.

Clearly, at this point the surgeon is entering into a conflict and is attempting to be confrontational, questioning your clinical competence and essentially side-lining you altogether. The important task here is to engage the surgeon in a professional, respectful manner.

"Dr. Smith, your patient's safety is my number one priority. This is not a matter of who is the clinician. We have a sick patient who appears to be having a worsening of symptoms. I assure you, this patient is at heightened risk for anesthesia, regardless of who the anesthesiologist is. The safest course for this patient is to have her return to her pulmonologist for optimization of her symptoms and once that occurs, we can proceed with the case."

Here, we begin with a neutralizing statement (your patient's safety is my number one priority). By starting with this statement, we are trying to align our goals with the surgeon's (patient safety). We now repeat what is already stated, but focus on the fact that safety will be compromised if the case moves ahead, even if the surgeon finds another anesthesiologist. Again, conflict resolution cannot be a moment to lose your own temper or, even worse, concede safety precautions to the surgeon. Rather, you must stand your ground and use medical concepts to justify your position.

This scenario more than the others is more about conflict resolution than anything else. Use of layperson's terms are not necessary here as you are speaking with another physician. However, focusing on complications and having a clear plan for how you believe the condition can be optimized will be key assets to doing well on this OSCE.

7 Clinical Scenario #6: Practice-Based Learning and Improvement

The hospital administrators are concerned about a lower than desired proportion of first case on-time starts in the main operating rooms. One of your colleagues, Dr. Jane Doe, has been tasked by the department chair to design and implement a quality improvement (QI) project to improve the proportion of cases starting on time. Dr. Doe has never conducted a QI project and has asked for your assistance. You have only a few minutes between cases available to talk, but Dr. Doe wants to get a general idea from you about the steps needed to perform a QI project.

Task Statement

Your task is to explain to your colleague the general steps of how to design and implement a QI project. The discussion should NOT focus on the specifics of on-time OR starts, but rather on your general approach to any QI project.

Action Plan

For this particular scenario, the ABA wishes to have the student complete the following tasks: (1) measure current outcomes and benchmarks, if appropriate; (2) devise change in practice in collaboration with stakeholders, if appropriate; (3) educate and train clinicians regarding change in practice as appropriate; (4) implement change in practice; and (5) measure outcomes after change in practice.

Step 1: Identify the Science of a QI Project

The basic premise of any QI project is that there is a certain negative outcome that is caused by a defect in the workflow. For perioperative medicine, that workflow often involves nurses, surgeons, and anesthesiologists.

To conduct a proper QI project the following five steps must be taken:

1. Identify the problem (late starts).
2. Collect data related to the problem.
3. Use the collected data to identify sources of errors that contribute to the problem.
4. Develop a corrective action plan.
5. Educate the necessary stakeholders on the corrective measures.

In this scenario, step #1 (identifying the problem) will have already taken place. Thus, our job here is to work through steps 2–5.

Step 2: Approach the Colleague

The board is very clear that they do not wish for this scenario to focus on the specific situation (late starts). Thus, the discussion should be broad based and your response positive.

> "Hi, Dr. Doe. It would be my pleasure to go over the basics of QI projects with you."

Step 3: Begin Completing Tasks

For task #1, begin by giving a broad yet informative description of benchmarks and outcomes, using different examples.

> "For any QI project, start by collecting data. Specifically, the data should focus on benchmarks and specific outcomes. For example, if the project was about patient satisfaction after surgery, then one of the outcomes you may wish to collect is their postoperative pain score, as this may be a cause of dissatisfaction. Also, in situations where the project is measuring, let's say, start time or turnover time, you may wish to collect when specific tasks were completed, such as when was the OR ready for the patient, when was the patient seen by the preoperative nurse, or when the surgeon had the patient sign the consent. Thus, before you do anything, you need to identify what information you think you will need in order to analyze the situation and begin collecting that data BEFORE any intervention."

The actor may challenge your statement. Consider this as an opportunity to further explain your logic.

> Actor: This seems very redundant. Isn't it better to just make some changes and see if it does anything?
>
> Student: Well, before you make changes, you need to know where you are starting from and what changes make the most sense. You do not want to change something that is working and potentially make the situation worse. For example, if you are initiating a QI project to improve patient satisfaction scores and, without any data collection, immediately started administering more pain meds to patients under the assumption that they were dissatisfied mainly because of pain, then you may not improve your satisfaction scores if postoperative pain was already adequately controlled and there were other, non-pain-related issues causing the overall dissatisfaction. Much worse, administering more pain medication can lead to undesirable side effects, which may cause your scores to drop further.

Thus, in these two statements, the student has adequately demonstrated that he or she understands the need for measuring benchmarks and outcomes and can defend that decision to his or her colleagues.

In completing task #2, the student must discuss change in practice.

"Once you have a good amount of preintervention data, you will analyze it to see where there are problems. For projects involving first case on-time start, you may see that patients are arriving at the hospital too late, or they are being registered too slowly, or there are insufficient nurses for all of the patients to do preop with them. For patient satisfaction, you may identify that many of these patients are being discharged without proper patient education materials or that the majority of the patients speak a language other than English but discharge instructions do not reflect this. Once you have analyzed the data, you must make a determination of where changes are necessary and which individuals need to make the changes (i.e., administrators, nurses, surgeons, anesthesiologists, etc.)."

For task #3, education is emphasized.

"Educating the stakeholders is very important. This should begin by meeting with the chiefs (nursing or surgeon or anesthesia) and, through them, communicating with the group at large. This way you are not overstepping your bounds and are working with the existing hierarchy to implement change. It is useful at this stage to present the data as well, so everyone is aware of what is occurring. You can also at this stage propose a "launch" date for the new process that you believe will improve the outcome."

Tasks #4 and #5 can be covered in one statement:

"Identifying the date for the change is essential because this way everyone involved knows a new process will be in place. Thus, everyone can be ready to be a part of the change and resistance is minimal. It is also important to collect data after the change is made so that you can compare the preintervention data to the postintervention data and potentially show the improvement in outcome."

The details of how to construct and execute a QI project are very basic. This should be an extremely simple OSCE to earn points in. However, it is important to practice discussing the five core steps involved in this process.

Index

INDEX

INDEX

www.ingramcontent.com/pod-product-compliance
Ingram Content Group UK Ltd.
Pitfield, Milton Keynes, MK11 3LW, UK
UKHW061617290626
13445UKWH00040B/888

9 780190 852474